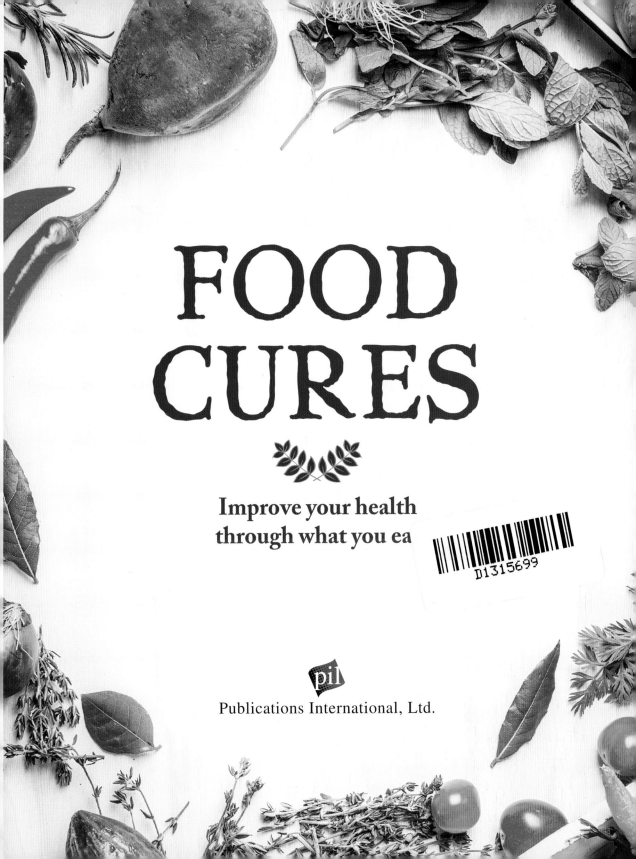

FOOD CURES

**Improve your health
through what you ea**

pil

Publications International, Ltd.

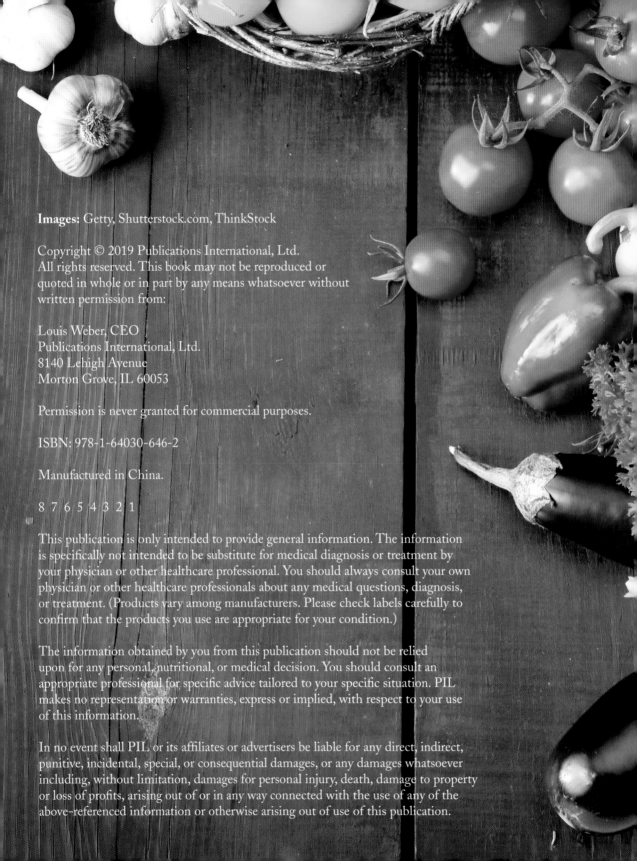

This publication is only intended to provide general information. The information
is specifically not intended to be substitute for medical diagnosis or treatment by
your physician or other healthcare professional. You should always consult your own
physician or other healthcare professionals about any medical questions, diagnosis,
or treatment. (Products vary among manufacturers. Please check labels carefully to
confirm that the products you use are appropriate for your condition.)

The information obtained by you from this publication should not be relied
upon for any personal, nutritional, or medical decision. You should consult an
appropriate professional for specific advice tailored to your specific situation. PIL
makes no representation or warranties, express or implied, with respect to your use
of this information.

In no event shall PIL or its affiliates or advertisers be liable for any direct, indirect,
punitive, incidental, special, or consequential damages, or any damages whatsoever
including, without limitation, damages for personal injury, death, damage to property
or loss of profits, arising out of or in any way connected with the use of any of the
above-referenced information or otherwise arising out of use of this publication.

TABLE OF CONTENTS

INTRODUCTION

Many of the most common health problems we face today—from annoying problems constipation to more serious conditions such as heart disease—are linked to what we eat. Within the last several decades, the focus of research into possible links between nutrition and health has expanded; it now includes not only the potential dangers of eating certain foods (or too much of certain foods) but also the natural healing and protective powers that some foods possess.

That's not to say that food alone can cure disease or take the place of medical treatment. It is, however, becoming increasingly evident that food has disease-fighting potential. Translation? You have the power to choose foods that may help prevent and treat a host of today's most common maladies.

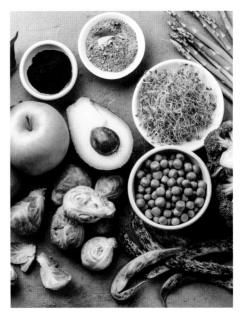

The more we research, the more proof we have: **Eating well and good health are intertwined.** Eating right can't prevent or cure every illness—but eating nutrient-dense foods that give us the vitamins and minerals we need is necessary for good long-term health. More than that, for a number of chronic conditions, including certain foods in your diet—or excluding others—can help soothe symptoms, forestall further health problems, and even reverse the progression of the disease.

In *Food Cures*, you will find information about how food interacts with more than fifty health conditions. Some, like colds and stomach upset, are short-term problems. What you eat during that time can help you ride out the unpleasantness and provide fast relief for symptoms. In other cases, for chronic conditions like diabetes and heart disease, your long-term food choices are critical to your management of the disease.

You may be surprised by how much what you eat affects seemingly unrelated health conditions. We understand intuitively how our diet can be used to treat symptoms of gallbladder disease or irritable bowel syndrome, for example, but not immediately see a link between our diet and Alzheimer's disease, or depression, or anxiety. Nonetheless, our food choices affect the health of our entire body, from our brain down to our feet. In *Food Cures*, you'll find out how. The book provides both concrete suggestions for specific foods that address specific conditions, along with recommendations for which vitamins and minerals you need more of.

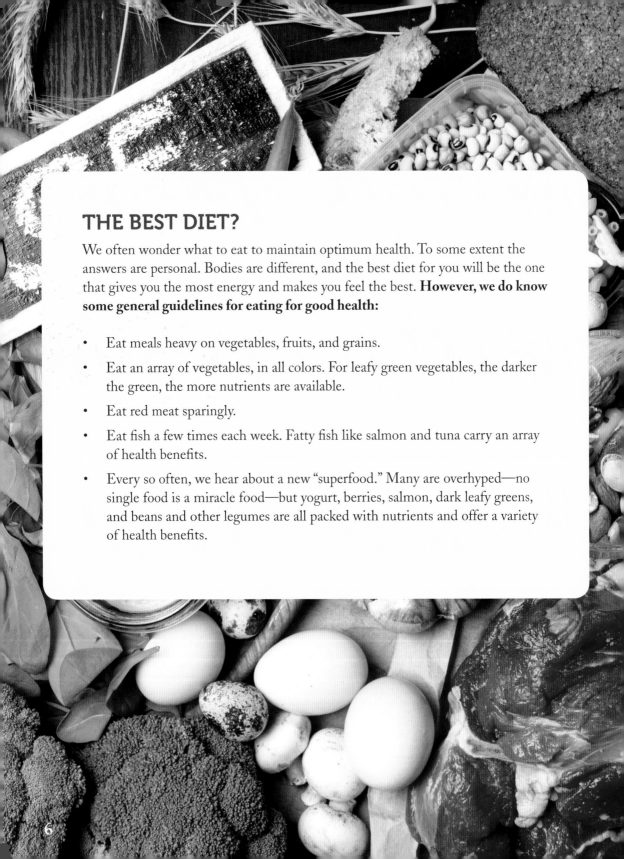

THE BEST DIET?

We often wonder what to eat to maintain optimum health. To some extent the answers are personal. Bodies are different, and the best diet for you will be the one that gives you the most energy and makes you feel the best. **However, we do know some general guidelines for eating for good health:**

- Eat meals heavy on vegetables, fruits, and grains.

- Eat an array of vegetables, in all colors. For leafy green vegetables, the darker the green, the more nutrients are available.

- Eat red meat sparingly.

- Eat fish a few times each week. Fatty fish like salmon and tuna carry an array of health benefits.

- Every so often, we hear about a new "superfood." Many are overhyped—no single food is a miracle food—but yogurt, berries, salmon, dark leafy greens, and beans and other legumes are all packed with nutrients and offer a variety of health benefits.

THE ROLE OF MULTIVITAMINS

Getting enough of essential nutrients is a good start on the road to a healthy immune system. And generally, eating a well-balanced diet will get you on that road. But you may be thinking about taking a multivitamin to help fill in the gaps. Are they worth it? And what should you look for? Most nutrition experts would tell you to get the majority of your nutrients from food—mostly because there are other good-for-you components in food that a specific vitamin may not offer. Taking a multivitamin is a good backup plan. **If you decide to take a multivitamin, follow these tips:**

- Look for a vitamin/mineral combination. You need vitamins and minerals to enhance your immune system, so be sure the product you choose has all you need.

- Don't use products that have more than 100 percent of the recommended daily allowance (RDA) or daily value (DV) of a nutrient. You're going to get most of your vitamins and minerals from your diet, so don't go overboard.

- Make sure your multivitamin meets your needs. If you need to boost your immune system, look for a multivitamin that has vitamin E, C, B6, and zinc.

- Check the expiration date. Multivitamins may not start smelling up the place after they expire, but they can lose their potency.

- Only take what is recommended. One a day is exactly what you should take. Don't double up on pills.

GETTING STARTED

When it comes to putting healing medicine in an easy-to-swallow package, Mother Nature has truly outdone science. Fortunately, science is catching on and gradually uncovering the many ways that food, especially food in its natural state, appears able to help the body heal and protect itself. With the aid of *Food Cures*, you can put that newly discovered knowledge to work for your own health's sake, with each food you choose and each bite you take.

ALLERGIES

Allergies can be called a haywire response of the immune system. Normally, the immune system guards against intruders it considers harmful to the body, such as certain viruses and bacteria. That's its job. However, in allergic people, the immune system goes a bit bonkers. It overreacts when you breathe, ingest, or touch a harmless substance. The benign culprits triggering the overreaction, such as dust, pet dander, and pollen, are called allergens.

The body's first line of defense against invaders includes the nose, mouth, eyes, lungs, and stomach. When the immune system reacts to an allergen, these body parts make great battle-grounds. Symptoms include runny nose; sneezing; watery, swollen, or red eyes; nasal conges-tion; wheezing; shortness of breath; a tight feeling in the chest; difficulty breathing; coughing; diarrhea; nausea; headache; fatigue; and a general feeling of misery. Symptoms can occur alone or in combination.

WHAT CAUSES ALLERGIES?

Blame your genes. The tendency to become allergic is inherited, and allergies typically de-velop before age 30. What you become allergic to is based on what substances you are exposed to and how often you are exposed to them. Generally, the more you are exposed to an aller-gen, the more likely it is to trigger a reaction.

Unfortunately, there is no cure for allergies. But there are ways to ease your long-suffering sinuses and skin, both in the short term and the long term.

FOODS TO BOOST THAT IMMUNE SYSTEM

An allergy-sufferer's hardworking immune system may increase demands for certain nutrients, both to protect the body and to help rebuild defenses. Be sure your diet includes the following vitamins and minerals:

- **Vitamin A.** If you eat a well-balanced diet, you should have an ample supply.
- **Vitamin B complex.** B vitamins are found in almost every food, but the best sources are from fresh vegetables and meats.
- **Vitamin C.** Citrus fruits are high in vitamin C.
- **Vitamin E.** High amounts are found in vegetable oils, nuts, and seeds. Moderate amounts are in avocados, asparagus, mangoes, apples, and sweet potatoes.
- **Iron.** The best sources are meats, oysters, whole grains (including hot cereals), beans, and green vegetables.

- **Selenium.** Find this mineral in meats, seafood, and whole grains.
- **Zinc.** Meats, oysters, dairy products, and some beans have good amounts of zinc.

KITCHEN CURES

BASIL. To help ease an allergic reaction or hives, try dousing the skin with basil tea, a traditional Chinese folk remedy. Basil contains high amounts of an anti-allergic compound called caffeic acid. Place 1 ounce dried basil leaves into 1 quart boiling water. Cover and let cool to room temperature. Use the tea as a rinse as often as needed.

MILK. Milk does the body good, especially when it comes to hives. Wet a cloth with cold milk and lay it on the affected area for 10 to 15 minutes. When it comes to drinking, though, pass up the milk. When allergies act up, skip that extra-large, whole-milk latte since dairy products thicken mucus.

TEA. Allergy sufferers throughout the centuries have turned to hot tea to provide relief for clogged-up noses and irritated mucous membranes. One of the best for symptom relief is mint tea, which has been used by the Chinese to treat allergies since the seventh century.

Mint's benefits extend well beyond its delicious smell. Mint's essential oils act as a decongestant, and substances within the mint contain anti-inflammatory and mild antibacterial constituents.

WASABI. If you're a hay fever sufferer and sushi lover combined, this remedy will please. Wasabi, that pale-green, fiery condiment served alongside California rolls, is a member of the horseradish family. Anyone who has taken too big a dollop of wasabi or plain old horseradish knows how it makes sinuses and tear ducts spring into action. That's because allyl isothiocyanate, a constituent in wasabi, promotes phlegm flow and has antiasthmatic properties. The tastiest way to get in those allyl isothiocyanates is by slathering horseradish on your sandwich or plopping wasabi onto your favorite sushi. The last, harder-to-swallow option is to purchase grated horseradish and take $1/4$ teaspoon during an allergy attack.

* TO MAKE * MINT TEA:

Place $1/2$ ounce dried mint leaves in a 1-quart jar. Fill two-thirds of the jar with boiling water and steep for five minutes (inhale the steam). Let cool, strain, sweeten if desired, and drink.

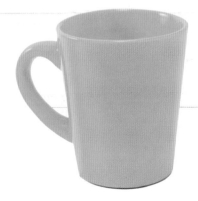

ALZHEIMER'S DISEASE

Alzheimer's disease (AD) is everyone's worst nightmare. Most diseases destroy either a physical or a mental function. Alzheimer's seizes both, slowly and steadily destroying memory, logical thought, and language. Simple tasks—how to eat or comb hair—are forgotten, and once AD sets in there's no turning back the clock.

The disease is named for Dr. Alois Alzheimer, a German doctor who, during an autopsy in 1906, discovered physical changes in the brain of a woman who had died of a strange mental illness. He found plaques and tangles in her brain, signs that are now considered hallmarks of AD.

A PROGRESSIVE DISEASE

AD is one of a group of brain disorders called dementia, which are progressive degenerative brain syndromes that affect memory, thinking, behavior, and emotion. Alzheimer's is the most common cause of dementia: Between 50 and 60 percent of all cases of dementia can be attributed to Alzheimer's.

Early symptoms include difficulty remembering names, places, or faces and trouble recalling things that just happened. Personality changes and confusion when driving a car or handling money are also early symptoms. Eventually mild forgetfulness progresses to problems in comprehension, speaking, reading, and writing. And physical breakdown occurs, too, partly because tasks such as eating and drinking are simply forgotten or too difficult to accomplish.

While we don't know the cause of AD yet, we do know that there are dietary and environmental factors. Heredity has also been studied as a possible cause.

Since we don't know what causes AD, we also do not yet have a cure for it. However, the picture is not as bleak as it was a decade ago. Research is turning up some remedies that can help alleviate symptoms as well as slow the advancement of the disease. And the good news is that many of these can be found right in your kitchen.

EASY EATING

Using utensils can become difficult for people with Alzheimer's, so solve the problem by offering finger foods. Keep them simple, handy, and nutritious.

Some suggestions:

- Fortified breads
- Peanut butter sandwiches
- Easy to grab fruits, such as bananas, apricots (especially dried apricots, which are high in potassium), peeled apple wedges (apple peels can cause choking), carrots, and celery sticks
- Chocolate-covered almonds or almond M&Ms. Almonds are rich in vitamin E, which may delay the progression of AD. Two ounces of almonds a day supplies the recommended amount of vitamin E.

KITCHEN CURES

ALMOND EXTRACT. This contains vitamin E. Try baking some almond cookies.

BLUEBERRIES. Evidence suggests they contain an antioxidant that may slow down age-related motor changes, such as those seen in Alzheimer's.

CARROTS. These are loaded with beta-carotene, which is a memory booster. Carrot and beet juice are good for the memory, too. So are okra and spinach.

CITRUS FRUITS. These fruits are loaded with vitamin C, which is believed to help protect brain nerves. Berries and some vegetables, including peppers, sweet potatoes, and green leafy vegetables, are also rich sources of vitamin C.

EGGS. It doesn't matter how you eat them. Eggs are loaded with vitamin A, which may protect brain cells and enhance brain function. Other vitamin A-rich foods include liver, spinach, milk, squash, and peaches.

FISH. Fatty acids, which AD sufferers often lack, are important in keeping those brain nerves healthy. Fish are high in fatty acids (that's why they're often called "brain food"), so it's a good idea to eat fish several times a week. Good choices include salmon, mackerel, sardines, and anchovies.

GINGER. This spice can stimulate a poor appetite. Try some ginger tea or gingersnaps, or chop up some fresh ginger and mix it with a little lime juice and a pinch of rock salt, then chew. It will not only increase appetite but thirst, too.

GREEN LEAFY VEGETABLES. These are high in folic acid, which may stimulate cognitive function. Other good sources of folic acid include beets, black-eyed peas and other legumes, Brussels sprouts, and whole-grain foods.

LEMON OIL. Steep a few drops of lemon or peppermint oil in hot water, then inhale. These are aromatherapy stimulants; they can perk up those suffering typical AD symptoms such as lethargy or depression.

MEAL SUPPLEMENTS. These meal-in-a-can beverages are easy to drink, and they're fortified with vitamins and minerals.

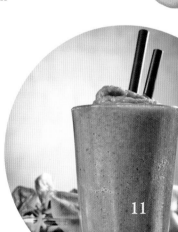

ORANGE JUICE. This is another way to up your vitamin C intake, but don't combine it with buffered aspirin. The two, taken together, form aluminum citrate, which is absorbed into the body five times faster than normal aluminum.

RED VEGETABLES. Research from the Netherlands suggests that people who eat large amounts of dark red, yellow, and green vegetables may reduce their risk of dementia by 25 percent.

SAGE. For depression associated with AD, drink a tea made with $1/2$ teaspoon sage and $1/4$ teaspoon basil steeped in 1 cup hot water twice a day.

SEEDS. Pumpkin, sesame, and sunflower seeds are packed with essential fatty acids necessary for brain function.

SESAME OIL. Depression associated with AD may be relieved with nose drops of warmed sesame oil. Use about 3 drops per nostril, twice a day.

SOY PRODUCTS. Studies suggest that isoflavones found in soy protein may protect postmenopausal women from AD. Try these: soy milk over cereal, soy meat substitutes, tofu frozen treats. And substitute tofu for ricotta or cream cheese in recipes. Dietary guidelines suggest 20 to 25 grams soy protein a day.

TURMERIC. Curcumin, an antioxidant and anti-inflammatory compound in this spice, has been found to reduce the number of plaques in the brain of mice and thus may slow the progression of Alzheimer's.

WHEAT GERM OR POWDERED MILK. Add to foods for extra protein.

MORE DO'S & DON'TS

- Don't serve foods with pits or bones.
- Always check food temperature. Hot and cold sensations can be numbed in people with AD, but they still can get burned.
- Don't serve foods with a mixture of textures. They may be hard to swallow.
- Serve foods that require little chewing, such as soups, ground meat, and applesauce.
- Serve several smaller meals instead of three main meals.
- Select favorite foods, especially if the appetite is poor. And keep in mind that as the disease progresses, food preferences may change.
- Play music at meals. Mealtimes can be stressful and music is relaxing. Choose songs from the patient's youth or that hold a special memory.

KITCHEN CAREGIVER CREATIVITY

Familiarity is important to those suffering with AD, and what is more familiar than the kitchen? It's a reminder of good things and good times, and even the easiest of kitchen tasks can stimulate memory as well as provide the activity that those with AD need every day. Here are some simple kitchen tasks to try that might trigger a wonderful memory.

These activities must be assisted:

- Clip coupons
- Fill the sugar bowl
- Peel carrots
- Fold kitchen towels
- Empty dishwasher

- Wipe off the table
- Organize silverware
- Set the table
- Make sandwiches
- Bake cookies

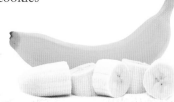

✳ BANANA ✳
BASICS

It's one of nature's true miracles, and for those with Alzheimer's, it's a nutritional miracle. One of the most common problems plaguing people with AD is low fluid intake. Those with the disease simply forget to drink, or they choose not to in order to avoid bathroom emergencies and accidents. The result is dehydration, which can cause a loss of potassium, which in turn, contributes to confusion. The simple solution for restoring essential potassium to the body is to force fluids—water or sports drinks with potassium—but that's often easier said than done. So the next best solution grows in bunches, is easy to eat, and tastes great.

Here are the banana facts you need to know:

- One ripe, medium-size banana supplies about 13 percent of the body's daily need for potassium.

- Bananas are a great source of fast energy. Very ripe bananas are loaded with sugar, about 23 grams, which is digested quickly and easily, then converted into energy. Ripe bananas are not recommended for people with diabetes.

- Bananas are easy to chew and swallow, which can be very important in AD since these functions may become impaired.

ANEMIA

Anemia is a condition in which your red blood cell count is so low that it can't carry enough oxygen to all parts of your body. Not having enough oxygen in the blood is like trying to drive a car with no oil. Your car may run for a while, but you'll soon end up with a burned-out engine. In the same way that oil nourishes your car's engine, oxygen provides needed nourishment for your body's tissues (organs, muscles, etc.), and if they aren't getting enough of that vital sustenance, you'll start feeling weak and tired. A short climb up the stairs will leave you breathless, and even a couple days of rest won't perk you up. If that describes how you feel, check with your doctor. If you do have anemia, you should take action as soon as possible. And you need to be sure you don't have a more serious condition.

ANATOMY OF ANEMIA

Your red blood cells are the delivery trucks of the body. They carry oxygen throughout your blood vessels and capillaries to feed tissues. Hemoglobin, the primary component of red blood cells, is a complex molecule and is the oxygen carrier of the red blood cell.

The body works very hard to ensure that it produces enough red blood cells to successfully carry oxygen but not too many, which can cause the blood to get too thick. Red blood cells live only 90 to 120 days. The liver and spleen get rid of the old cells, though the iron in the cells is recycled and sent back to the marrow to produce new cells.

When you're diagnosed with anemia it usually means your red blood cell count is abnormally low, so it can't carry enough oxygen to all parts of your body, or that there is a reduction in the hemoglobin content of your red blood cells. Anemia is not a disease in itself but instead is considered a condition. However, this condition can be a symptom of a more serious illness. That's why it's always important to check with your doctor if you think you may be anemic.

THE MOST COMMON CAUSES OF ANEMIA

There are many types of anemia. Some rare types are the result of a malfunction in the body, such as early destruction of red blood cells (hemolytic anemia), a hereditary structural defect of red blood cells (sickle cell anemia), or an inability to make or use hemoglobin (sideroblastic anemia). The most common forms of anemia are the result of some type of nutritional deficiency and can often be treated easily with some help from the kitchen.

These common types are:

• Iron deficiency anemia. Iron deficiency anemia happens when the body doesn't have enough iron to produce hemoglobin, causing the red blood cells to shrink. And if there's not enough hemoglobin produced, the body's tissues don't get the nourishing oxygen they need. Children younger than three years of age and premenopausal women are at highest risk for developing iron deficiency anemia. Most young children simply don't get enough iron in their diet, while heavy menstrual periods are the most common cause of iron deficiency anemia in women who are pre-menopausal. In addition, during pregnancy a woman's blood volume increases three times, boosting iron needs. Contrary to popular belief, men and older women aren't at greater risk for iron deficiency anemia. If they do end up developing the condition, it's most often the result of an ulcer.

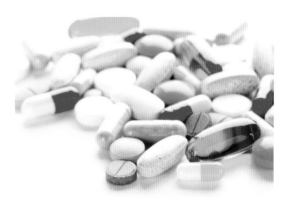

• Vitamin B12 deficiency anemia. While iron deficiency anemia produces smaller than usual red blood cells, a vitamin B12 deficiency anemia produces oversized red blood cells. This makes it harder for the body to squeeze the red blood cells through vessels and veins. It's like trying to squeeze a marble through a straw. Vitamin B12-deficient red blood cells also tend to die off more quickly than normal cells. Most people get at least the minimum amount of B12 that they need by eating a varied diet. If you are a vegetarian or have greatly limited your intake of meat, milk, and eggs for other health reasons, you may not get enough of the vitamin in your diet. Many older people are more at risk for vitamin B12 deficiency; in fact, 1 out of 100 people older than 60 years of age are diagnosed with pernicious anemia. This age group is at increased risk because they are more likely to have conditions that affect the body's ability to absorb vitamin B12. Surgical removal of portions of the stomach or small intestine; atrophic gastritis, a condition that causes the stomach lining to thin; and diseases such as Crohn's can all interfere with the body's ability to absorb vitamin B12. But the most common cause of vitamin B12 deficiency anemia is a lack of a protein called intrinsic factor. Intrinsic factor is normally secreted by the stomach; its job is to help vitamin B12. Without intrinsic factor, the vitamin B12 that you consume in your diet just floats out as waste. In some people, a genetic defect causes the body to stop producing intrinsic factor. In other people, an autoimmune reaction, in which the body mistakenly attacks stomach cells that produce the protein, results in a lack of intrinsic factor. A vitamin B12 deficiency that is caused by a lack of intrinsic factor is called pernicious anemia. Pernicious anemia can be particularly dangerous because it causes neurological problems, such as difficulty walking, poor concentration, depression, memory loss, and irritability. These can usually be reversed if the condition is treated in time. Unfortunately, in the case of pernicious anemia, the stomach cannot absorb the vitamin no matter how much B12-rich food you eat. So treatment requires injections of B12, usually once a month, that bypass the stomach and shoot the vitamin directly into the bloodstream.

• Folic acid deficiency anemia. A deficiency of folic acid produces the same oversized red blood cells as a vitamin B12 deficiency. One of the most common causes of folic acid deficiency anemia is simply not getting enough in the diet. The body doesn't store up folic acid for long periods like it does many other nutrients, so if you aren't getting enough in your diet, you will quickly become deficient. Pregnant women are most at risk for folic acid anemia because the need for folic acid increases by two-thirds during pregnancy. Adequate folic acid intake is essential from the start of pregnancy because it protects against spinal defects in the fetus.

IRON'S ASBORPTION EQUATION

You may not be absorbing as much iron from your foods as you think. How much you absorb is dependent on two primary factors: what kind of iron is in the food and what other nutrients the food contains. There are two types of iron, heme and non-heme. Heme, found primarily in foods of animal origin, is much more easily absorbed than non-heme iron, which is found primarily in plant products. But if you eat a vitamin C-rich food or a food rich in heme iron with your non-heme iron food, your body will take in more iron.

Here's a guide to top iron sources:

- **Sources of mostly heme iron:** beef liver, lean sirloin, lean ground beef, skinless chicken, pork

- **Sources of non-heme iron:** fortified breakfast cereal, pumpkin seeds, bran, spinach

- **Sources of vitamin B12:** salmon, beef tenderloin, yogurt, shrimp

- **Sources of folic acid:** spinach, navy beans, wheat germ, avocado, orange

KITCHEN CURES

BLACKSTRAP MOLASSES. Consider covering that waffle or those pancakes in a little molasses. Blackstrap molasses has long been known to be a nutritional powerhouse. Containing 3.5 mg of iron per tablespoon, blackstrap molasses has been used in folk medicine as a "blood builder" for centuries.

DRY CEREAL. Fix yourself a bowl of your favorite cereal (go for one without the sugar and the cartoon characters on the box), and you'll be waging a battle against anemia. These days many cereals are fortified with a nutrient punch of iron, vitamin B12, and folic acid. Check the label for amounts per serving, pour some milk over your flakes, and dig in.

BEEF LIVER. Beef liver is rich in iron and all the B vitamins (including B12 and folic acid). In fact, beef liver contains more iron per serving—5.8 mg per 3 ounces—than any other food. Other animal sources of iron include eggs, cheese, fish, lean sirloin, lean ground beef, and chicken.

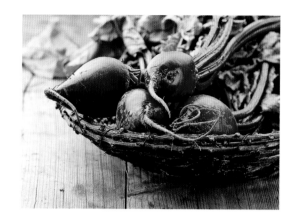

BEETS. Beets are rich in folic acid, as well as many other nutrients, such as fiber and potassium. The best way to prepare beets is to nuke 'em in the microwave. Keep the skin on when cooking, but peel before eating. The most nutrient-dense part of the beet is right under the skin.

SPINACH. Green leafy vegetables contain loads of iron and folic acid. We're talking dark and green, so choose your leaves carefully. Iceberg lettuce is mostly water and is of little nutritive value. Spinach, on the other hand, has 3.2 mg of iron and 130 mcg of folic acid per 1/2 cup.

MORE DO'S AND DON'TS

- If you're a vegetarian or have cut way down on your intake of meats, milk, and eggs, be sure that you're getting adequate amounts of iron and vitamin B12 in your diet. With such a diet, you are at greater risk for nutritional deficiency anemias because iron from plant sources isn't absorbed as well as iron from animal sources and because vitamin B12 is found almost exclusively in animal foods.

- Eat foods rich in vitamin C at the same time that you eat whole grains, spinach, and legumes, in order to increase absorption of the iron they contain.

- If you drink coffee or tea, do so between meals rather than with meals, because the caffeine in these beverages reduces iron absorption.

ANXIETY

Anxiety is a feeling everyone experiences sooner or later. Perhaps you're sitting in the waiting room, anticipating the horse-size needle your doctor has waiting for you on the other side of the door. Or you've spent all day cooking but the look on your mother-in-law's face says your best efforts were wasted. Or you really hate your job.

These very different experiences can bring on anxiety and its typical symptoms:

- heart palpitations
- sense of impending doom
- inability to concentrate
- muscle tension
- dry mouth
- sweating
- queasy, jittery feeling in the pit of the stomach
- hyperventilation

Anxiety can be short- or long-lived, depending on its source. The more long lasting the anxiety, the more additional symptoms you will experience.

If your anxiety is a reaction to a single, isolated event—the shot the doctor is about to give you—your anxiety level will decrease and your symptoms will disappear after the event. If your anxiety is from friction between you and your mother-in-law, you're likely to experience anxiety for a period of time before and after you see her. In this case, the symptom list may have grown to include diarrhea or constipation and irritability.

Then there's that job, a source of anxiety that never leaves you. You dread getting up in the morning because you have to go to work, dread going to bed at night because when you wake up you have to go to work, dread the weekend because when it's over you'll have to go to work. When the source of your anxiety is ever-present, you can probably add the following to the list of symptoms: chest pain, over- or under-eating, insomnia, loss of sex drive.

All three situations described above are types of everyday anxiety, or as some would put it, the cost of living. But the cost can be huge, taking its toll on you physically, mentally, and emotionally.

While emotion is most often at the root of anxiety symptoms, they can be caused by physical problems as well. **Rule out the following causes before assuming your symptoms are stress-related:**

- Hyperthyroidism, which may produce symptoms that resemble those of anxiety
- Heart disorders, which can cause rapid heartbeat, often associated with anxiety. If you experience chest pain, numbness, shortness of breath, or dizziness, call your doctor or 9-1-1 immediately.
- Caffeine, which can produce nervous symptoms even in moderate amounts
- Premenstrual syndrome (PMS)
- Diet pills
- Anemia
- Diabetes
- Hypoglycemia

So now that you know what anxiety can do, it's time to learn what you can do to control it. Mild anxiety can be often treated successfully at home with a little calming music, a little quiet time, and some soothing remedies from the kitchen.

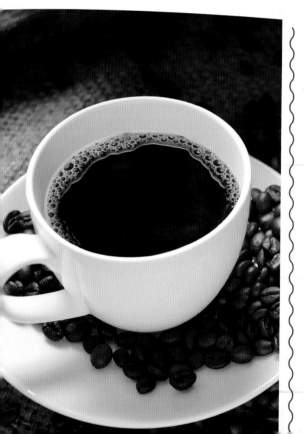

* TIPS ON CUTTING THE CAFFEINE

Because caffeine can cause anxiety, and caffeine addiction symptoms mimic anxiety, this good-morning pick-me-up is at the head of the no-no list. But cutting it out all at once can cause withdrawal symptoms, including anxiety, irritability, headache, and fatigue.

To stop, cut back gradually until you are caffeine free and have no withdrawal symptoms. If you do experience withdrawal symptoms, especially as you near the end of all caffeine consumption, continue drinking 1 cup of a caffeinated beverage daily, then gradually cut back on that.

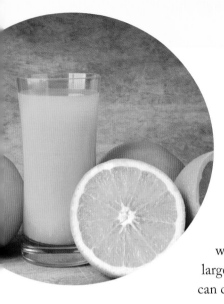

KITCHEN CURES

ALMONDS. Soak 10 raw almonds overnight in water to soften, then peel off the skins. Put almonds in blender with 1 cup warm milk, a pinch of ginger, and a pinch of nutmeg. Drink at night to relax you before going to bed.

CELERY. This Hoosier remedy may calm your nerves. Eat 2 cups celery, onions, or a mixture of the two, raw or cooked, with your meals for a week or two. Both vegetables contain large amounts of potassium and folic acid, deficiencies of which can cause nervousness.

ORANGE. The aroma of an orange is known to reduce anxiety. All you have to do to get the benefits is peel an orange and inhale. You can also drop the peel into a small pan or potpourri burner. Cover with water and simmer. When heated, the orange peel will release its fragrant and calming oil.

ORANGE JUICE. For a "giddyap" heart rate associated with anxiety, stir 1 teaspoon honey and a pinch of nutmeg into 1 cup orange juice and drink.

ROSEMARY. Once used by early Californians to rid them of "evil spirits," rosemary has a calming effect on the nerves. Make a tea by adding 1 to 2 teaspoons of the dried herb to 1 cup boiling water; steep for 10 minutes, then drink. Inhaling rosemary can be relaxing, too. Burn a sprig, or use rosemary incense to ease anxiety.

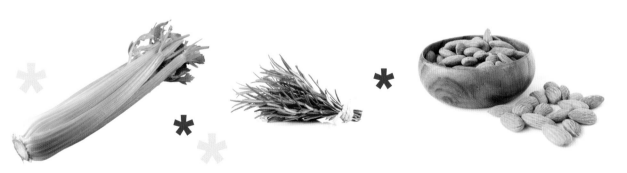

TOO MUCH ENERGY?

Studies indicate that the release of lactate into the blood may cause anxiety. Alcohol, caffeine, and sugar are all lactate culprits. A deficiency in the B vitamins niacin and thiamin, as well as in omega-3 fatty acids and calcium, can contribute to anxiety.

NIACIN-RICH FOODS	THIAMIN-RICH FOODS	CALCIUM-RICH FOODS
liver	whole-wheat products	almonds
red meats	legumes	broccoli
fish	wheat germ	cottage cheese
yeast extracts	bran	milk
peanuts	eggs	salmon
legumes	whole-grain rice	yogurt
dried fruits		

FOLK REMEDY HERBAL CURES

These may not be found in your kitchen supplies, but if you experience frequent anxiety, it might be wise to give them an honored place of their own in the cupboard or drawer.

Warning! If you are taking any medication, whether it's over-the counter or prescription, do not use any herbal remedy without first consulting your doctor. These cures can have bad side effects when mixed with other drugs!

Catnip. You may keep this one around for Fluffy, but it can help alleviate human anxiety. Make a tea by steeping 3 teaspoons catnip in 1 cup boiling water for 10 minutes. Sweeten to taste and drink three times a day.

Chamomile. This calms the nerves and aids in getting to sleep, and the taste isn't bad as herbal cures go. When you feel anxious, brew a cup of chamomile tea. Simply steep 1 tablespoon chamomile flowers in 1 cup water for 15 minutes, then strain and drink as needed. Breathe in its aroma, too, for a soothing effect. Use chamomile in an aroma lamp, sachet, or potpourri. However, since chamomile contains pollen, be careful if you have allergies.

Ginseng. Simmer the root on low heat in enough water to cover the root twice. When half the water is evaporated, remove from heat to cool. Strain and drink twice a day. You can also buy ginseng extracts that readily dissolve in hot water.

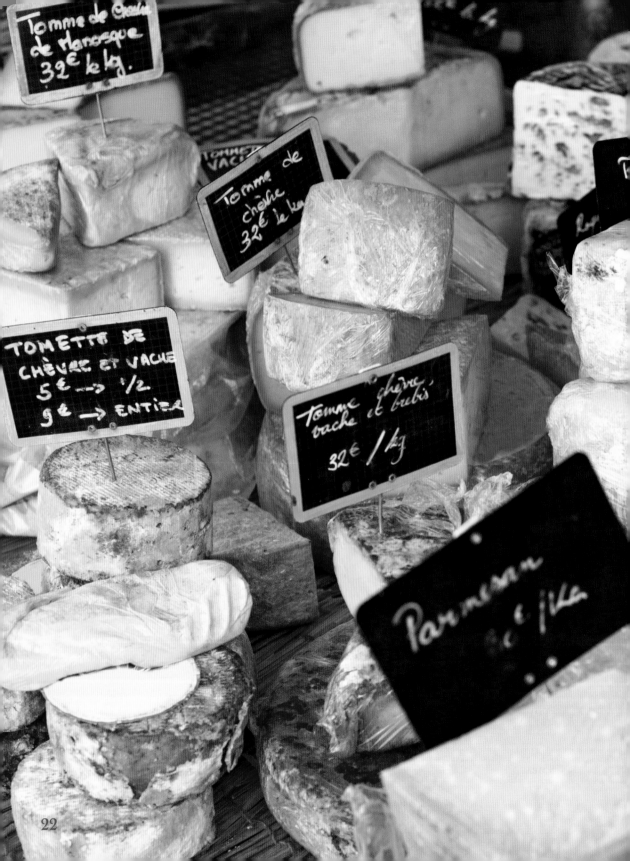

Tomme de Chèvre
de Manosque
32€ le kg.

Tomme de
chèvre
32€ le kg

TOMETTE DE
CHÈVRE ET VACHE
5€ --> 1/2
9€ --> ENTIER

Tomme de chèvre,
vache et brebis
32€ / kg

Parmesan
€/kg

22

ARTHRITIS

Arthritis means inflammation of the joints. To the millions of Americans afflicted by one of the 100 varieties of arthritis, every day can be painful. The two most prevalent forms of arthritis are osteoarthritis and rheumatoid arthritis.

Osteoarthritis (OA), the most common form, is the result of joint cartilage wearing down over time. When the durable, elastic tissue is gone, bones rub directly against one another. This causes stiffness and dull pain in the weight-bearing joints (hips, knees, and spine) and in the hands. The elderly are most susceptible to OA, but athletes and those in jobs requiring repetitive movements are also very vulnerable.

Rheumatoid arthritis (RA) is the inflammation of the joint lining. The cause is unknown, but it is thought that the symptoms are the result of the body turning against itself. Symptoms of RA vary from individual to individual. In its mildest form, it causes minor joint discomfort. More often, however, the inflammation causes painful, stiff, swollen joints, and in prolonged cases, severe joint damage. Unlike OA, whose symptoms are joint-specific, RA tends to cause body-wide symptoms such as fatigue, fever, and weight loss.

While it's typically thought that old age puts one at risk for arthritis, this isn't the case with RA. RA usually develops between the ages of 20 and 50 and is more common in women than in men.

Waking up with a stiff back or swollen finger joint doesn't necessarily indicate arthritis; however, should pain, stiffness, or swelling last more than two weeks, you may have arthritis. **Other symptoms include:**

- Swelling in one or more joints
- Early morning stiffness
- Recurring pain or tenderness in a joint
- Inability to move a joint in a normal fashion
- Redness or warmth in a joint
- Unexplained weight loss, fever, or weakness accompanied by joint pain

There is no cure for arthritis, but many kitchen-crafted remedies can help ease the pain.

KITCHEN CURES

DAIRY PRODUCTS. Some medicines used to treat arthritis can lead to a loss of calcium from the bones, resulting in osteoporosis. To counteract this effect (and to keep healthy in general) make sure you get enough calcium in your diet. A cup of low-fat yogurt, for instance, supplies 300 to 400 mg calcium—about one-third of your daily requirement. Calcium-fortified orange juice will also help you meet your daily calcium needs.

GAMMA LINOLENIC ACID. Recent research suggests that high doses of an omega-6 essential fatty acid, known as gamma linolenic acid (GLA), can help reduce joint inflammation. You'll find GLA in some plant seed oils, such as evening primrose and borage, and in black currants. Research also indicates that the benefits of GLA may be enhanced by supplementation with omega-3 fatty acids, which are plentiful in cold-water fish. You can also take GLA supplements; 1,800 mg a day is recommended for rheumatoid arthritis.

SUPPLEMENTS

CALCIUM. The Recommended Daily Allowance is 1,000 mg calcium per day for women prior to menopause and 1,200 to 1,500 mg after menopause. Men require 800 mg per day. If you don't get enough calcium in your diet, be sure to supplement to protect your bones.

GLUCOSAMINE. Glucosamine supplements, often found in products that contain a combination with chondroitin, help relieve the pain and may slow the joint degeneration associated with osteoarthritis. The recommended dosage is 500 mg of glucosamine three times a day. It usually takes two to three months of supplementation for maximum benefit.

TRACK WHAT WORKS

Decreasing arthritis pain and stiffness may be as easy as eliminating certain foods from your refrigerator and, thus, from your diet. However, the deduction process is a bit difficult, requiring time and observation. There are no set guidelines for this remedy. Rather, it is intuitive. Do you ache more after eating a certain food? Keep a food diary, record what you've eliminated from your diet that week, and rate your discomfort level. There are no guarantees, but you may discover that certain foods contribute to stiffness.

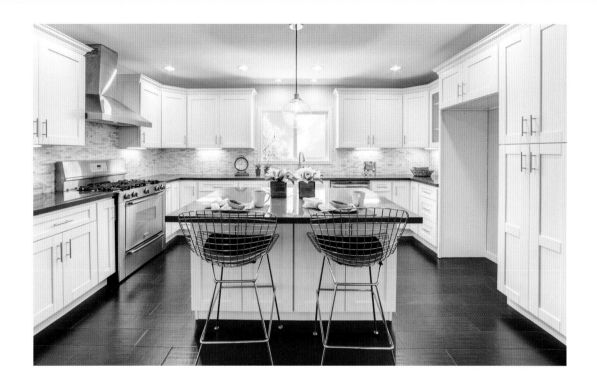

SETTING UP YOUR KITCHEN

Little adjustments in the kitchen itself may make a big difference in protecting arthritic joints from injury or excessive strain.

- Buy kitchen drawer knobs with long, thin handles. These require a looser, less stressful grip.

- More padding, less pain. On tools that require a grip, such as mops and brooms, tape a layer of thin foam rubber around the handles and fasten with tape.

- Use lightweight pots and pans with comfortable handles.

- Utilize a pair of long-handled pinchers (or a gripper) to pick up objects on the floor.

- Transport groceries or heavy items from car to kitchen using a wagon or cart.

- Use loops made of soft, strong fabric to pull the refrigerator and oven doors open without strain.

ASTHMA

Asthma is the number one cause of chronic illness in kids, affecting more than 5.5 million children. Despite this discouraging news, there is reason to be hopeful if you are one of the millions of asthmatics across the country. As the numbers of asthma cases continue to climb, researchers are even more determined to find asthma's causes and develop more effective treatments.

BREATHING BASICS

When you take a breath, the air goes from your mouth or nose to the windpipe (or trachea). It then travels to the lungs. It first enters the lungs through the bronchi, a group of tubes that branch off from the windpipe. The bronchi then branch off into bronchioles. Imagine a car driving from the interstate to a state highway to a country road and you get the picture. Asthma happens when the bronchi and bronchioles come in contact with a foreign invader, or asthma "trigger." There are many different triggers, and each person has his own set. Once a foreign material enters the body, the airways quickly become inflamed, causing the muscles that rest on the outside of the airways to tighten and narrow. This allows a thick mucus to enter the airways. The mucus causes swelling and makes it very difficult to breathe. The classic symptoms of an asthma attack include wheezing, tightening in the chest, dry coughing, and increased heart rate. These are frightening symptoms to experience, and they're also quite alarming for someone to observe.

Though there are many natural ways to help asthma sufferers breathe easier, experts recommend that combining certain natural remedies with prescription anti-inflammatories and bronchodilators are your best bet to attack your asthma.

KITCHEN CURES

COFFEE. The caffeine in regular coffee can help prevent and treat asthma attacks. Researchers have found that regular coffee drinkers have one-third fewer asthma symptoms than those who don't drink the hot stuff. And caffeine has bronchodilating effects. In fact, caffeine was one of the main anti-asthmatic drugs during the nineteenth century. Don't load up on java, though. Three cups a day will provide the maximum benefit.

CHILI PEPPERS. Hot foods such as chili peppers open up airways. Experts believe this happens because peppers stimulate fluids in the mouth, throat, and lungs. The increase in fluids thins out the mucus formed during an asthma attack so it can be coughed up, making breathing easier. Capsaicin, the stuff that makes hot peppers hot, acts as an anti-inflammatory when eaten and a bronchodilator when inhaled in small doses.

ONIONS. Onions are loaded with anti-inflammatory properties. Studies have shown that these properties can reduce the constriction of the airways in an asthma attack. Use cooked onions, as raw onions are generally too irritating.

ORANGE JUICE. Vitamin C is the main antioxidant in the lining of the bronchi and bronchioles. Research discovered that people with asthma had low levels of vitamin C and that eating foods that had at least 300 mg of vitamin C a day—equivalent to about 3 glasses of orange juice—cut wheezing by 30 percent. Other foods high in vitamin C include red bell pepper, papaya, broccoli, blueberries, and strawberries.

SALMON. Fatty fish such as sardines, salmon, mackerel, and tuna contain omega-3 fatty acids. These fatty acids seem to help the lungs react better to irritants in people who have asthma and may even help prevent asthma in people who have never had an attack. Studies have found that kids who eat fish more than once a week have one-third the chance of getting asthma as children who don't eat fish. And researchers discovered that people who took fish oil supplements, equivalent to eating 8 ounces of mackerel a day, increased their body's ability to avoid a severe asthma attack by 50 percent.

YOGURT. Vitamin B12 can improve the symptoms of asthma and seems to be even more effective in asthma sufferers who are sensitive to sulfite. Studies have found that taking 1 to 4 micrograms (mcg) works best as protection against asthma attacks.

✳ FOODS TO AVOID

Some asthma sufferers are particularly sensitive to the chemical preservatives sulfites. Sulfites are found in many kinds of foods and beverages. If you have a question about a food, check out the label. Sulfites will probably be listed among the ingredients. Here are some common foods with high concentrations of sulfites:

- Wine
- Lemon juice
- Dried fruits
- Fresh shrimp
- Instant potatoes
- Canned veggies
- Fruit topping
- Molasses
- Wine vinegar
- Corn syrup
- Pizza dough
- Grapes
- Beer
- Instant tea

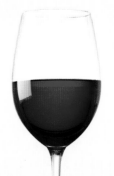

BACK PAIN

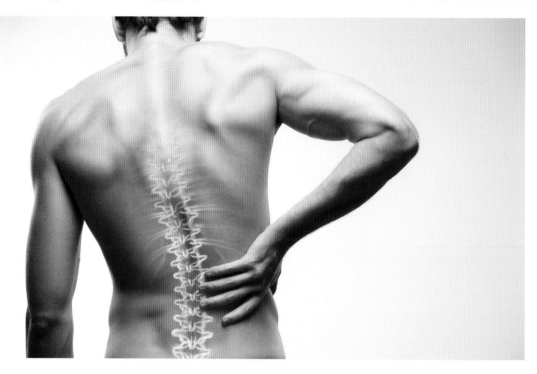

People are bad to their backs, crouching over keyboards for eight hours, struggling to lift heavy objects, or quickly transforming themselves from sedentary office workers to weekend warriors. Whatever the action, the back often can't handle such stress, and it reacts with pain.

Almost everyone will experience back pain once in their life. Lower back pain has many causes, including common muscle strain and more serious problems with the bones in the spine (vertebrae) and the disks of shock-absorbing material that separate them. Why is the lower back such a glutton for punishment? Unlike the upper back, it isn't supported by the rib cage, and many people don't exercise the back and the supporting abdominal muscles as they should.

Back pain remedies rely primarily on rest, strengthening and stretching exercises, and modification of daily routine. However, the kitchen shelves do hold a few ingredients that can help get that back back into shape.

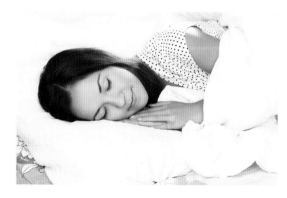

KITCHEN CURES

CHAMOMILE TEA. Daily stress can turn back muscles into a knot. Luckily, chamomile tea offers some calming relief to soothe tense muscle tissue. During a break or after work, treat yourself to a steaming mug. Steep 1 tablespoon chamomile flowers in 1 cup boiling water for 15 minutes. Or, you can use a prepackaged chamomile tea. Drink 1 to 3 cups a day.

Warning! Chamomile contains allergy-inducing proteins related to ragweed pollen. Ask your doctor about drinking chamomile if you are allergic to ragweed. Packaged tea may be safer to drink than tea made from the flowers. Your doctor can advise you.

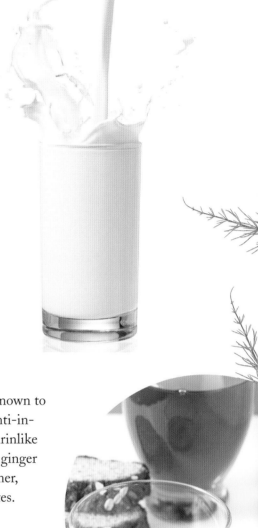

GINGER ROOT. Fragrant ginger root has long been known to cure nausea, but back pain, too? Ginger does contain anti-inflammatory compounds, including some with mild aspirinlike effects. When your back aches, cut a 1- to 2-inch fresh ginger root into slices and place in 1 quart boiling water. Simmer, covered, for 30 minutes on low heat. Cool for 30 minutes. Strain, sweeten with honey (to taste), and drink.

MILK. Bone up on milk. Women especially should take care to include plenty of calcium in their diets. (Older women are at greater risk for developing osteoporosis, the disease of eroding bones.) Calcium helps build strong bones and protect the spine from osteoporosis.

ROSEMARY. Rosemary's leaves are packed with these anti-inflammatory substances: carnosol, oleanolic acid, rosmarinic acid, and ursolic acid, all of which work to ease swollen tissues. To make a pain-relieving tea: Place $1/2$ ounce dried rosemary leaves into 1 quart boiling water. Cover and steep for 30 minutes. Drink 1 cup tea at bedtime and another cup before eating breakfast.

BELCHING

It's not a big deal, not even a medical condition most of the time. It's simply the result of swallowing air. But the air that goes down has to go somewhere, so most of the time it leaves the same way it came in—through the mouth. We all belch. Even the most prim of the proper is not exempt from this oftentimes untimely eruption.

Belching does serve a purpose other than embarrassment, however. It removes gas from the stomach by forcing it up into the esophagus and then on out your mouth. Without this escape device, we'd blow up like a big balloon, not to mention the sharp cramps we'd feel running all the way from our stomach to our throats. So belching is a good thing. And no matter how many good ones we let out during the course of a day, the swallowed air that turns into a burp is only a tiny fraction of the intestinal gas that we all have.

THE CAUSE

Swallowing air, which is called aerophagia, is the primary offender when it comes to producing a belch. **We swallow air all the time, especially when we:**

- Eat and drink
- Talk
- Yawn and sigh
- Breathe through the mouth
- Smoke
- Chew gum or suck on hard candy

Here are some other reasons we belch:

- Belching occurs when we eat because food in the belly displaces the air that was already swallowed and is sitting in the stomach.
- Anxiety is a cause of belching, too. We get nervous, we swallow more air. The more nervous we are, the more air we swallow, and the more we belch. Anxiety belching is usually habitual and subconscious. We swallow air into the esophagus and expel it before it hits the stomach.
- An improper denture fit can cause you to swallow air.
- Drinking carbonated beverages.
- Excessive swallowing due to postnasal drip.
- Although belching is not normally a symptom of illness, some gastrointestinal disorders are accompanied by belching, including gallstones, hiatal hernia, ulcer, and gastritis.

Even with all the conditions belching could potentially indicate, most often belching is simply belching for the sake of letting out unneeded gasses.

Medically, belching is called eructation. Of course, that occasional and inadvertent little burp may slip out, and often at the most embarrassing moment. If its escape is, indeed, occasional, there's nothing to worry about. But if it happens more often than you'd like, you can look to your kitchen for a cure.

KITCHEN CURES

CARAWAY. Try some caraway seeds, straight or sprinkled on a salad. They calm the digestive tract.

CUMIN. Roast equal amounts of cumin, fennel, and celery seed. Combine. After you eat, chew well about ¹/₂ to 1 teaspoon of the mixture, then chase it down with ¹/₃ cup of warm water.

DILL SEED TEA. Drop 1 teaspoon dill seeds into 1 cup boiling water, then steep for 15 minutes. Strain, then drink. Try the same with fennel or chamomile.

GINGER. Ginger tea can help relieve the need to belch. Pour 1 cup boiling water over 1 teaspoon freshly grated gingerroot. Steep for 5 minutes, then drink.

LEMON JUICE. This works whether it's fresh or from the bottle. Mix 1 teaspoon lemon juice with ¹/₂ teaspoon baking soda in 1 cup cool water. Drink it quickly after meals.

PAPAYA. Most cures for belching aren't found in the fridge. But there is one surefire belch begone in the fruit drawer: papaya! It's full of an enzyme called papain that can get rid of whatever's causing that burp.

PEPPERMINT. Pour 1 cup boiling water over 1 teaspoon dried mint. Steep for five minutes.

YOGURT. Eat some yogurt with live cultures (check the label) every day. It aids digestion.

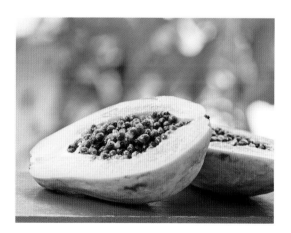

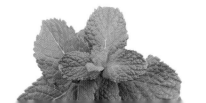

BRONCHITIS

That nasty cold has been hanging on much longer than it should, and day by day it seems to be getting worse. Your chest hurts, you gurgle when you breathe, and you're coughing so much yellow, green, or grey mucus that your throat is raw. These symptoms are letting you know that your cold has probably turned into a respiratory infection called bronchitis, an inflammation of the little branches and tubes of your windpipe that also makes them swell. No wonder breathing has become such a chore. Your air passages are too puffy to carry air very easily.

Acute bronchitis can include these other symptoms, too:

- Wheezing
- Shortness of breath
- Fever or chills
- General aches and pains
- Upper chest pain

Bronchitis is not contagious since it's a secondary infection that develops when your immune system is weakened by a cold or the flu. Some people are prone to developing it, some are not. Those at the top of the risk list have respiratory problems already, such as asthma, allergies, and emphysema. People who have a weakened immune system also are more prone to bronchitis. But anyone can develop it, and most people do at one time or another.

Under most circumstances, bronchitis will go away on its own once the primary infection is cured. But in those few days when you have it, it can sure be miserable. Here are a few kitchen tips that can relieve some of the symptoms.

KITCHEN CURES

ALMONDS. These little cure-all nuts have loads of vitamins and nutrients, and they are reputed to help everything from mental acuity to sexual vitality. Rich in potassium, calcium, and magnesium, almonds are especially known for their healing powers in respiratory illness. So when you're down with bronchitis, eat them in any form, except candy-coated or chocolate-covered. Sliver some almonds and garnish your veggies. They're also good in a citrus fruit salad for a little added crunch or rubbed in a little honey, coated with cinnamon, and roasted in a 325°F oven for 10 to 25 minutes.

ANISEED. Here's a bronchitis cough reliever that's also said to relieve heartburn. Boil 1 quart water, then add 7 teaspoons aniseed. Simmer until the water is half gone, strain the seeds, and add 4 teaspoons each of honey and glycerine (glycerine is available at the drugstore). Take 2 teaspoons every few hours.

BAY LEAF. Ancient Romans and Greeks loved bay leaves. They believed that this simple herb was the source of happiness, clairvoyance, and artistic inspiration. Whatever the case, it does act as an expectorant and is best taken in tea. To make the tea, tear a leaf (fresh or dried) and steep in 1 cup boiling water. **Warning!** Bay leaf tea should not be used during pregnancy, as it may bring on menstruation. Another bronchitis remedy with bay leaf is to soak some leaves in hot water and apply as a poultice to the chest. Cover with a kitchen towel. As it cools, rewarm.

COFFEE. The xanthine derivatives in coffee are good bronchodilators. To cut down on mucus problems, add 1 teaspoon apple cider vinegar and 2 drops peppermint oil to a cup of black coffee, either instant or brewed. Drink 1 cup in the morning and evening.

GINGER. This is a potent expectorant that works well in tea. Steep $1/2$ teaspoon ginger, a pinch of ground cloves, and a pinch of cinnamon in 1 cup boiling water.

HONEY. To relieve the cough that comes from bronchitis, slice an onion into a bowl, then cover with honey. Allow to stand overnight, then remove the onion. Take 1 teaspoon of the honey four times a day.

HORSERADISH. The irritating allyl isothiocyanates (mustard derivatives) in horseradish open up the sinuses. Be careful not to use horseradish if you're having stomach problems, though, because it's too potent.

Eat it straight, on a salad, or atop meat. Fresh horseradish is the best choice, but commercial products will work, too. Make sure it's straight horseradish, though. Sandwich spreads with horseradish won't work.

LEMONS. These help rid the respiratory system of bacteria and mucus. Make a cup of lemon tea by grating 1 teaspoon lemon rind and adding it to 1 cup boiling water. Steep for five minutes. Or, you can boil a lemon wedge. Strain into a cup and drink. For a sore throat that comes from coughing, add 1 teaspoon lemon juice to 1 cup warm water and gargle. This helps bring up phlegm.

ONIONS. These are expectorants and help the flow of mucus. Use raw, cooked, baked, in soups and stews, as seasoning, or any which way you like them.

SAVORY. This potent, peppery herb is said to rid the lungs of mucus. Use it as a tea by adding $1/2$ teaspoon savory to 1 cup boiling water. Drink only once a day.

THYME. This herb helps rid the body of mucus, strengthens the lungs to fight off infection, and acts as a shield against bacteria. Use it dried as a seasoning or make a tea by adding $1/4$ to $1/2$ teaspoon thyme (it's a very strong herb, so you don't need much) to 1 cup boiling water. Steep for 5 minutes and sweeten with honey. If you have thyme oil on hand, dilute it (2 parts olive or corn oil to 1 part thyme oil) and rub on the chest to cure congestion.

MUCUS-MAKERS TO AVOID

When you're congested, there are a few simple foods that should be avoided because they produce more mucus. **Here's the list:**

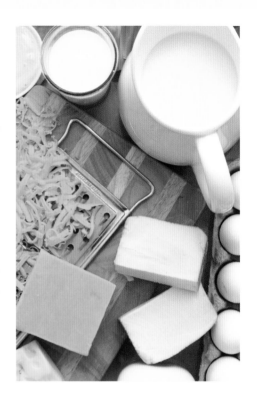

- Dairy foods
- Sugary products, including carbonated and noncarbonated soft drinks; sugar-coated cereal; sugary throat lozenges
- Refined cereals, bread, pasta
- Fried and fatty foods
- Red meat, including pork

    Here's a handy avoidance reminder:
    When you're congested, skip the white stuff—milk, flour, sugar.

BRONCHITIS-FRIENDLY FOODS

These won't cure, but studies indicate that foods rich in these nutrients may protect against another bout of bronchitis. The more vegetables you eat, the more protection you have.

BETA CAROTENE	VITAMIN E	VITAMIN	OMEGA-3 FATTY ACIDS
carrots	avocados	mackerel	herring
sweet potatoes	green leafy veggies	canned red salmon	kippers
apricots	whole-grain cereal	anchovies	mackerel
mangoes		whole milk	salmon
green veggies		cheese	sardines
		egg yolks	trout
			fresh tuna
			crab

BURSITIS

You head out to the backyard after a long winter indoors to turn over your garden. Later that day, you feel an unfamiliar pain in your shoulder. The dull ache becomes a more intense pain, and you start to think you might be getting arthritis. Because it causes pain and stiffness near the joint, many people mistake bursitis for arthritis. But bursitis is a different problem altogether. It can hit any major joint, including the shoulder, elbow, hip, ankle, heel, or base of the big toe.

BURSITIS BASICS

Bursa are tiny sacks of fluid that protect your muscles and tendons from rubbing against the rough edges of your bones. There are 150 bursa in your body, and any one of them can become inflamed. Inflamed bursa are very painful.

Most cases of bursitis clear up in a couple weeks if you stop aggravating the area, but there are some nutritional secrets that may help prevent future bursitis flare-ups.

KITCHEN CURES

ORANGE JUICE. Vitamin C is a wonder nutrient. Its antioxidant properties make it an ideal addition to the diet, especially when you are recovering from an injury. Vitamin C is vital for preventing and repairing injuries. Not getting enough vitamin C has been found to hinder proper formation and maintenance of bursa. Men and women older than 15 years of age need at least 60 milligrams a day. Drink just ³/₄ cup orange juice a day and you've met your daily quota.

PINEAPPLE. Pineapples contain bromelain, an enzyme that studies have shown reduces inflammation in sports injuries, such as bursitis, and reduces swelling.

TURMERIC. Studies have found that turmeric, specifically the yellow pigment in turmeric called curcumin, is a very effective anti-inflammatory. In animal studies turmeric was as effective as cortisone, and it didn't have any side effects.

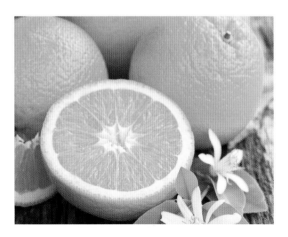

CANKER SORES

That wonderful spaghetti sauce has been simmering on the burner for hours, and you can't wait for the feast to begin. Just one last taste before culinary paradise and...Zap! It got you. It stings and your eyes tear up just a bit. All your well-planned preparations have been conquered by a painful canker, squelched by stomatitis (an inflammation of the mouth), annihilated by an apthous ulcer (the medical name for a canker).

Cankers are small white sores with red edges that develop inside your mouth. They hurt like the dickens, but usually they're not serious. The most painful phase lasts about three to four days, and the sores go away in about ten days. More than 80 percent of all mouth sores are cankers, but many people confuse them with cold sores (fever blisters), which they are not. Canker sores, unfortunately, can be repeaters, and some people are simply predisposed to getting them over and over. Most of the time the sores are not a major concern. They usually don't get infected, spread, or bleed if you don't bite them. But they're definitely a major pain. You can find over-the-counter antiseptic creams, lozenges, and mouthwashes at your local pharmacy to help relieve canker sore pain. But you can also find some relief over the kitchen counter in some common and not so common kitchen staples.

KITCHEN CURES

CRANBERRY JUICE. Drink this juice between meals: It's both a pain reliever and canker healer.

HONEY. Mix 1 teaspoon honey with ¼ teaspoon turmeric and dab it on your canker. This one may sting a bit.

SAGE. Used most often to spice up turkey stuffing, this herb is one that can be used to calm an angry canker. Simply add 3 teaspoons sage leaves to 1 pint boiling water. Steep, covered, for 15 minutes. Rinse your mouth with the liquid several times a day. You can also rub sage leaves into a powder and apply them directly to your sore.

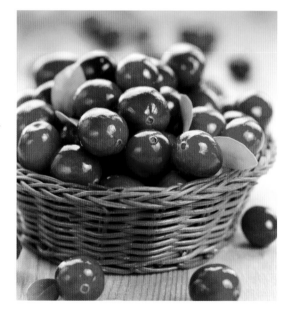

TEA. Moisten a regular tea bag and apply it directly to the canker. The tannic acid will help dry it out.

VITAMINS AND MINERALS

Deficiencies in vitamins and minerals are suspected of being a cause of canker sores. Make sure you get enough of these minerals in your diet by checking out the food chart below, or considering a supplement that contains the RDAs of both.

Because a nutritional deficiency, particularly in vitamin B12 and minerals iron and zinc, is suspected as a cause of canker sores, it's a good plan to eat foods that are rich in those vitamins and minerals. Try to include some of each of these foods in your diet to help ward off canker sores.

IRON	B12	FOLIC ACID	ZINC
• Meat • Fish • Poultry • Nuts • Seeds • Green leafy vegetables	• Liver • Meat • Poultry • Fish • Dairy products	• Beets • Green leafy vegetables • Black-eyed peas & other legumes • Brussels sprouts • Whole-grain foods	• Oysters • Other shellfish • Red meats • Whole-grain cereals

 # EDIBLE NO-NOS

Some of canker's prevailing causes are said to be spicy, sour, or acidic foods. If you develop a canker after eating pineapple or a mild sandwich that you spiced up with mustard or barbecue sauce, these could be trigger foods. Only you know what you eat before cankers pop up, so if you're plagued and can't figure out why, keep a canker sore diary. Note the foods you eat before a canker erupts and also record other facts in your life such as menstrual cycle or hormonal fluctuations, medications you took, and undue stress. You may see a pattern. In the meantime, here are a few of the foods to avoid when that canker comes calling:

- Carbonated soft drinks
- Tomatoes and tomato-based products
- Citrus fruits
- Pineapple
- Spicy foods
- Foods at a hot temperature
- Chocolate
- **Foods with sharp edges:** crackers, chips
- Alcoholic beverages

COLDS

Every year Americans will suffer through more than one billion colds. That's one billion runny noses, coughs, sneezes, aches, and sore throats. Colds make such frequent appearances that the infection has come to be known as the "common cold."

Small children are the most likely to catch a cold: Most kids will have six to ten colds a year. That's because their young immune systems combined with the germy confines of school and day-care situations make them prime targets for the virus. The upside of having so many colds as a child is that you develop immunities to some of the 200 viruses that cause colds. As a result, adults get an average of only two to four colds a year. By the time most people reach age 60, they're down to about one cold per year. Women, however, especially women between 20 and 30 years old, get more colds than men.

HOW DO COLDS BEAT A PATH TO YOUR DOOR?

Viruses are like the bully that torments all the kids on the playground. After entering the mucous layer of your nose and throat, the cold virus strong-arms your cells until they let the virus take over, forcing the cells to produce thousands of new virus particles.

But the virus is not the reason your throat begins throbbing and your nose starts flowing like Niagara Falls. Your immune system is responsible for that. As the virus begins replicating, the body gets the message that it's time to go into battle. The little soldiers of the body, the white blood cells, run to the body's rescue. One of the weapons the white blood cells use in their virus war are immune system chemicals called kinins. During the battle the kinins tell the body to go into defensive mode. So that runny nose is really your body fighting back against the cursed virus. That should make you feel a little better while you lie on the couch surrounded by tissues.

Because there are so many viruses that cause colds, the exact virus that you contracted is not easily pinned down. The most likely culprit in most colds is a rhinovirus (rhino is a Greek word meaning "nose"). There are over 110 specific rhinoviruses, and they are behind 30 to 35 percent of most colds. The second most common reason for that aching head is a coronavirus. These are especially common in adults. An unknown viral assailant causes 30 to 50 percent of colds, and about 10 to 15 percent of colds are caused by a virus that will probably lead to something more serious, such as the flu.

HOW COLDS ARE SPREAD

The cold virus can take many routes to its ultimate destination—your cells. Most people are contagious a day before and two to four days after their symptoms start. **There are typically three ways a cold virus is spread:**

- Touching someone who has the virus on them. The virus can live for three hours on skin.

- Touching something that contains the virus. Cold viruses can live three hours on objects.

- Inhaling the virus through airborne transmission. It may sound implausible, but if someone sitting next to you sneezes while you are inhaling, voilà! It's likely you'll get a cold.

One study found that kids tend to get colds from more direct contact while adults tend to get colds from airborne viruses (moms of young children can expect to get colds both ways). Research has also found that emotional stress, allergies that affect the nasal passages or throat, and menstrual cycles may make you more susceptible to catching a cold.

WHERE'S THE COLD VACCINE?

Good question! One of the main reasons we don't yet have a vaccine for the cold is that they're just too hard to pin down. Viruses live inside cells, which means they are protected from most medicines in the bloodstream. So even if you took an antiviral drug, chances are your body wouldn't allow it to penetrate the cells. Another reason viruses are so difficult to kill is that they don't grow well in a laboratory setting. Their ultimate playground is a cool, dry place, just like the inside of your nose.

Don't give up hope, though. Researchers are still on the job. Scientists have discovered the receptor sites that the rhinovirus attaches to when it invades a cell. They tested an antibody that blocked these receptor sites and helped slow down the time the virus actually took to develop into a cold. It also reduced the severity of its symptoms.

A HEALING HERB

Echinacea's immune-stimulating properties have been proved in European tests. A favorite in folk medicine for centuries, echinacea is used in contemporary herbal treatments in Britain, Australia, and the United States. In Germany, where herbs are prescribed just like pharmaceutical medicines, this handy herb is prescribed for colds. German clinical tests have shown that echinacea can help decrease cold symptoms. For the best results, take echinacea at the onset of cold symptoms—but not for longer than two weeks.

While colds are here to stay for now, you don't have to be totally at their mercy. Thankfully, there are some things you can do to fend off the germs that cause colds, as well as techniques to ease your symptoms once you're sick.

KITCHEN CURES

CHICKEN SOUP. Science actually backs up what your mom knew all along—chicken soup does help a cold. Scientists believe it's the fumes in the soup that release the mucus in your nose and help your body better fight against its viral invaders. Chicken soup also contains cysteines, which are good at thinning mucus. And the soup provides easily absorbed nutrients.

CORN SYRUP. You can make a sugar-water gargle to ease your throat. Use 1 tablespoon syrup per 8 ounces warm water, mix together, and gargle.

HONEY. Make your own cough syrup by mixing together $1/4$ cup honey and $1/4$ cup apple cider vinegar. Pour the mixture into a jar or bottle and seal tightly. Shake well before using. Take 1 tablespoon every four hours.

PEPPERS. Hot and spicy foods are notorious for making your nose run and your eyes water. The hot stuff in peppers is called capsaicin and is pharmacologically similar to guaifenesin, an expectorant found in some over-the-counter cough syrups. This similarity leads some experts to believe that eating

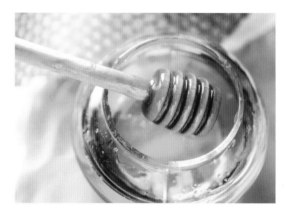

hot foods can clear up mucus and ease that stuffy nose.

TEA. A cup of hot tea with honey does the same trick as chicken soup; it loosens up your nasal passages and makes that stuffy nose feel better. Folk healers have known this secret for centuries. They often suggest drinking tea with spices and herbs that contain aromatic oils with antiviral properties. Try tea with elder, ginger, yarrow, mint, thyme, horsemint, bee balm, lemon balm, catnip, garlic, onions, or mustard.

YOGURT. One study found that participants who ate $3/4$ cup yogurt a day before and during cold season had 25 percent fewer colds. But you've got to start early and maintain your yogurt eating throughout the peak cold season.

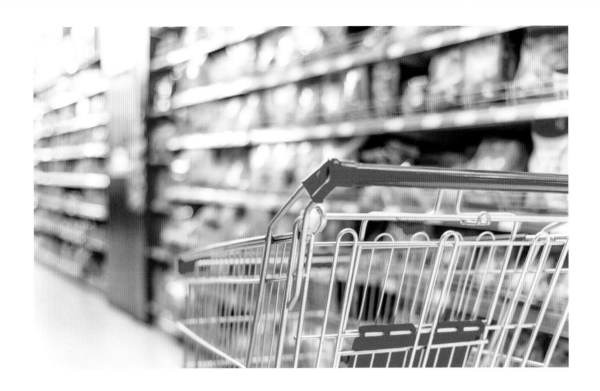

FROM THE SUPPLEMENT SHELF

VITAMIN C. Vitamin C won't prevent a cold, but research shows that it can help reduce the length and severity of symptoms. But to reap the benefits, you've got to take a lot of "C." The RDA for men and women 15 and older is 60 mg, but studies show that you'd need to take upward of 1,000 mg to 3,000 mg to get the cold-symptom-sparing rewards of vitamin C. For the short term, experts believe that wouldn't be harmful, but taking too much vitamin C for too long can cause severe diarrhea. Before loading up on vitamin C, check with your doctor.

ZINC. Studies have found that zinc may help immune cells fight a cold and may ease cold symptoms. The most effective zinc lozenges are those that contain 15 to 25 mg of zinc gluconate or zinc gluconate-glycine per lozenge. You can get the most out of your zinc lozenges if you start using them at the first sign of a cold and continue taking them for several days.

COLD SORES

You know it's coming when you feel that notorious tingling on your lip and the accompanying itching and burning. You can't help stressing out about it; all you can think about is the pain and embarrassment those ugly cold sores cause. But there's not a darned thing you can do to stop a cold sore, also known as a fever blister, from erupting.

Many people get confused about whether they have a cold sore or a canker sore. But that confusion is easily cleared up. If the sore is on your external lip or near your mouth or nose and looks like a fluid-filled blister, chances are it's a cold sore. Caused by a virus called herpes simplex Type 1, herpes blisters are very contagious. They also love company, so where there's one there are usually many. Within a few days to a week, the blisters break, ooze, and form an ugly yellow crust that can stay around for weeks. When it finally sloughs off, though, there's nice, healthy pink skin underneath. Best of all, cold sores leave no scars.

You can't cure cold sores, and they like to keep coming back, usually to the scene of a previous visit. When a cold sore's not making itself a huge lip ache, it's snoozing in the nerves below your skin, just waiting for a reason to wake up.

And what sets off its alarm clock?

- Fever
- Infection, colds, flu
- Ultraviolet radiation, such as a sunburn
- Stress
- Fatigue
- Changes in the immune system
- Trauma
- Food allergies
- Menstruation
- Dental work

Conventional medicine does have a few tricks in its little black bag, including antiviral lotions and creams. But they don't cure, just treat. So take a look in your kitchen. You might just find some useful treatments there, too.

KITCHEN CURES

LICORICE. Studies show that glycyrrhizic acid, an ingredient in licorice, stops the cold sore virus cells dead in their tracks. So try chewing a licorice whip. Just be sure it's made from real licorice, as most candy in the United States today is flavored with anise. If the ingredient list says "licorice mass," the product contains real licorice.

MILK. This remedy doesn't involve drinking. Soak a cotton ball in milk and apply it to the sore to relieve pain. Better yet, if you feel the tell-tale tingling before the cold sore surfaces, go straight to the cold milk. It can help speed the healing right from the beginning.

FOODS THAT FIGHT COLD SORES

There's a good amino acid, lysine, that helps block the herpes virus. **So try some foods high in this cold sore warrior, such as:**

- Meats
- Milk
- Fish
- Chicken
- Eggs
- Beans & bean sprouts
- Cheese

Foods rich in bioflavonoids can help prevent or speed up the course of the blisters that flare up, too. **These include:**

- Onions
- Apples
- Grapes
- Tea

Foods packed with vitamin C are also valiant in their quest to rid you of your herpes foe. **Eat a lot of these foods that are rich in vitamin C:**

- Oranges, grapefruits, seedless berries (they all make great smoothies)
- Peppers
- Green leafy vegetables
- Sweet potatoes and potatoes

✳ FOODS TO AVOID

During a herpes simplex episode, anything with arginine, an amino acid, is on the no-no list. Arginine causes the herpes virus to multiply. **Arginine-containing foods include:**

- Chocolate
- Peanuts and other nuts
- Raisins
- Seeds
- Wheat and wheat products
- Oats
- Coconut
- Soy beans

Several foods that don't contain arginine can also make the episode worse. Stay away from sugar, coffee, fried foods, and alcohol. If you're prone to cold sores, stay away from tobacco, too, as it suppresses the immune system. Skip spices and spicy foods. That includes taking a pass on mustard and barbecue. Watch the acidic fruits, too, such as oranges, grapefruits, and especially pineapples.

COLIC

Bringing home a newborn baby is one of life's greatest joys. Yet it can also be one of life's greatest trials, especially if that cute little bundle of joy cries constantly. That's the number one symptom of colic: nonstop crying combined with bouts of irritability and fussiness that last a total of more than three hours a day on more than three days of the week. Colic, if it happens, typically begins at around two weeks of age and tapers off around three months. It generally is more pronounced during the evenings. Parents will be pleased to know that despite the crying, most colicky babies are healthy, well-fed infants, and the condition isn't life threatening or classified as a disease.

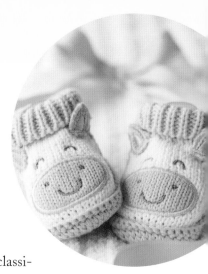

IT'S A MYSTERY

Unfortunately for both baby and parents, doctors don't know what causes colic, what the disorder is, or how to cure it. They don't even know if colicky babies are in pain. Fortunately for everyone involved, there are many tried-and-true ways to soothe a baby. Experiment with a few, determine what works, and stick to it.

KITCHEN CURES

BASIL. This aromatic herb contains large amounts of eugenol, which, among other things, has antispasmodic and sedative properties. Place 1 teaspoon dried basil leaves in a cup and fill it with boiling water. Cover and let stand for ten minutes. Strain and, while warm or at room temperature, give it to the infant in a bottle. A nursing mother may also drink the tea.

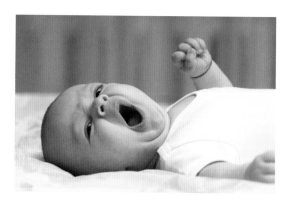

CHAMOMILE TEA. Chamomile combines antispasmodic and sedative properties and may relieve intestinal cramping and induce relaxation at the same time. In fact, chamomile contains 19 different antispasmodic constituents, as well as 5 sedative ones. To make a cup of tea: Place 1 teaspoon chamomile flowers in a cup and fill with boiling water. Cover and let stand for ten minutes. Strain and, while warm or at room temperature, give to the infant in a bottle. A nursing mother may also drink the tea, unless she is allergic to pollens. Prepackaged chamomile tea bags may be used instead of flowers.

MINT. Mint has antispasmodic properties, which may help reduce intestinal spasms in colicky infants. Place 1 teaspoon dried mint in a cup and fill with boiling water. Let stand for ten minutes. Strain well and, while warm, feed to the baby in a bottle. Nursing mothers may want to have a cup of mint tea, too. A peppermint stick soaked in water may be used as an alternative, but note that many sticks contain sugar. Never use straight peppermint oil to make tea. It's too potent for a baby.

SOY PRODUCTS. That carton of cow's milk looks innocent enough, but it can be the problem source for five to ten percent of colicky babies. Many studies have shown an improvement in colic after dairy products have been eliminated from babies' diets. The culprit seems to be the protein in cow's milk. (Don't think milk is the only villain. This protein lurks in many infant formulas containing dairy and is also found in the milk of breast-feeding mothers who consume dairy products.) Try eliminating dairy products for two weeks and switch to soy products, both for baby and for you if you're breast-feeding. If you don't notice any improvement, assume milk isn't the culprit.

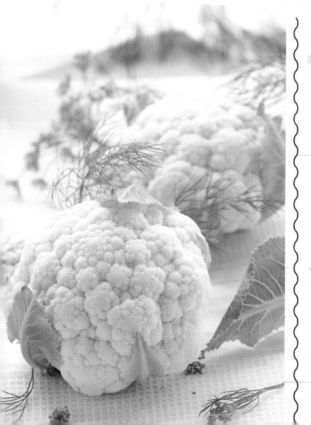

* WATCH
* WHAT **YOU EAT**

Many experts suggest nursing mothers look to recent dietary changes for the cause of colic. **Nursing mothers should try to avoid eating the following:**

- Garlic
- Onions
- Broccoli
- Cauliflower
- Cabbage
- Peanut butter
- Fish

If colic persists, avoid dairy foods and grains.

CONSTIPATION

Nothing's moving, even though you know you have to move your bowels. Everything in your body is sending you that signal. You feel bloated and uncomfortable pressure, but when you try to go, nothing happens. Or, if you do finally go, it hurts.

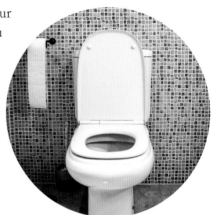

Constipation occurs for many different reasons. Stress, lack of exercise, certain medications, artificial sweeteners, and a diet that's lacking fiber or fluids can each be the culprit. Certain medical conditions such as an underactive thyroid, irritable bowel syndrome, diabetes, and cancer also can cause constipation. Even age is a factor. The older we get, the more prone we are to the problem.

And constipation is a problem, although it's not an illness. It's simply what happens when bowel movements are delayed, compacted, and difficult to pass.

WHAT'S NORMAL?

Some people mistakenly believe they must have a certain number of bowel movements a day or a week or else they are constipated. That couldn't be further from the truth, although it's a common misconception. What constitutes "normal" is individual and can vary from three bowel movements a day to three a week. You'll know if you're constipated because you'll be straining a lot in the bathroom, you'll produce unusually hard stools, and you'll feel gassy and bloated.

LAXATIVES AREN'T NUMBER ONE

It's not a good idea to use laxatives as the first line of attack when you're constipated. They can become habit-forming to the point that they damage your colon. Some laxatives inhibit the effectiveness of medications you're already taking, and there are laxatives that cause inflammation to the lining of the intestine.

Conventional thinking on laxatives is that if you must take one, find one that's psyllium- or fiber-based. Psyllium is a natural fiber that's much more gentle on the system than ingredients in many of the other products available today. Or, simply look in the kitchen for relief. It's there.

KITCHEN CURES

APPLES. Eat an hour after a meal to prevent constipation. In addition, apple juice and apple cider are natural laxatives for many people. Drink up and enjoy!

BANANAS. These may relieve constipation. Try eating two ripe bananas between meals. Avoid green bananas because they're constipating.

BARLEY. It can relieve constipation as well as keep you regular, and it has cholesterol-lowering properties, too. What more could you ask of a simple grain? Buy some barley flour, flakes, and grits. Add some barley grain to vegetable soup or stew.

BLACKSTRAP MOLASSES. Take 2 table-spoons before going to bed. It has a pretty strong taste, so you may want to add it to milk, fruit juice, or for an extra-powerful laxative punch, prune juice.

GARLIC. In the raw, it has a laxative effect for many. Eat it mixed with onion, raw or cooked, and with milk or yogurt for best results.

HONEY. This is a very mild laxative. Try taking 1 tablespoon three times a day, either by itself or mixed into warm water. If it doesn't work on its own, you may have to pep it up by mixing it half and half with black-strap molasses.

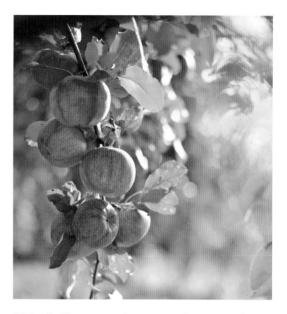

OIL. Safflower, soybean, or other vegetable oil can be just the cure you need, as they have a lubricating action in the intestines. Take 2 to 3 tablespoons a day until the problem is gone. If you don't like taking it straight, mix the oil with herbs and lemon juice or vinegar to use as salad dressing. The combination of the oil and the fiber from the salad ought to fix you right up.

PRUNES. Yep, they work! And here's a great-tasting way to cure constipation. Cover several prunes with boiling water. If you wish to sweeten the prunes, stir 1 or 2 teaspoons honey into the boiling water before you pour it over the fruit. Let the prunes stand in the water overnight, and eat them the next day. Drink the prune juice, too. This works with figs, as well.

RAISINS. Eat a handful daily, an hour after a meal.

RHUBARB. This is a natural laxative. Cook it and eat it sweetened with honey or bake it in a pie. Or, create a drink with cooked, pureed rhubarb, apple juice, and honey.

SESAME SEED. These provide roughage and bulk, and they soften the contents of the intestines, which makes elimination easier. Eat no more than $1/2$ ounce daily, and drink lots of water as you take the seeds. You may also sprinkle them on salads and other foods, but again, no more than $1/2$ ounce. Sesame is also available in a butter or paste and in Middle Eastern dips, such as tahini.

VINEGAR. Mix 1 teaspoon apple cider vinegar and 1 teaspoon honey in a glass of water and drink.

WALNUTS. Fresh from the shell, they may be just the laxative you need.

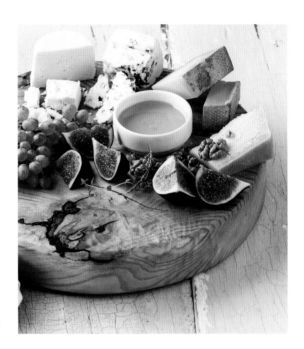

HERBAL REMEDIES

You won't necessarily find these in the kitchen cupboard, but if you do, they can help cure that constipation.

Flaxseeds. These provide natural bulk and will relieve constipation. Wash 2 teaspoons seeds in cold water. Add to 1 cup boiling water. Let steep for ten minutes, then drink. Do not strain out the seeds.

Senna. This will work, but children under 12 and women who are pregnant should not use it. Here's the recipe: Place $1/4$ to $1/2$ teaspoon crushed senna leaves or powder in 1 cup boiling water. Let it steep for ten minutes. Use once a day for no more than ten days.

Warning! Use only a small amount of senna. It's very strong, and one full teaspoonful can cause abdominal cramping.

COUGH

Annoying, loud, and disruptive, a persistent cough can put a damper on your daily routine. Coughs can be defined by how long they last. A brief cough is caused by such factors as cold air, irritating fumes, breathing dust, or drawing food into the airways. A persistent cough, however, typically results from mucus and other secretions brought on by respiratory disorders such as the cold, the flu, pneumonia, or tuberculosis.

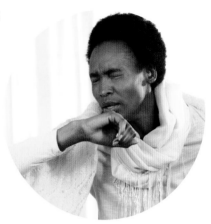

Moisture content also differentiates coughs. Some are dry, accompanied by a ticklish or sore throat. Others are accompanied by a thick phlegm and are called wet coughs.

A BENEFICIAL REFLEX

Regardless of time and moisture content, a cough is produced when viruses, bacteria, dust, pollen, or other foreign substances irritate respiratory passages in the throat and lungs. The cough reflex is the body's effort to rid the passageways of such intruders, and it spares no power in the expulsion. A cough reflex can expel a foreign substance at velocities as high as 100 miles per hour.

Determine what kind of cough you have and search out cures specific to that type. Some remedies aim to moisten dry throats, while others are expectorants, helping you cough up and get rid of mucus and irritants. Most of these kitchen cures aim to battle both coughs unless otherwise noted.

KITCHEN CURES

CHICKEN SOUP. Take some advice from your grandma: Sip a bowl of chicken soup. It doesn't matter if it's homemade or canned. Chicken soup is calming for coughs associated with colds. While scientists can't put a finger on why this comfort food benefits the cold sufferer, they do believe chicken soup contains anti-inflammatory properties that help prevent a cold's miserable side effects, one being the cough. Plus, chicken soup contains cystein, which thins phlegm. The broth keeps you hydrated, and it all tastes yummy.

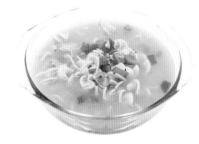

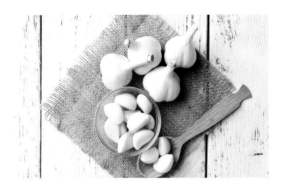

GARLIC. Eating garlic won't have you winning any kissing contests, but who wants to kiss you when you sound like a seal? Since kissing isn't on your agenda, you can indulge in one of nature's best cures for coughs: garlic. It's full of antibiotic and antiviral properties, plus garlic is also an expectorant, so it helps you cough up stubborn bacteria and/or mucus that are languishing in your lungs.

Some experts advise that to reap garlic's full cold- and flu-fighting benefits, you have to eat it raw. Yet swallowing 4 to 8 raw garlic cloves a day (the recommended amount) is hard for most people to stomach. Cheat a little by mixing the cloves into plain yogurt and putting a dollop on your soup. If you make a pasta sauce, put the garlic in at the last moment, or toss garlic slices into your salad.

A cup of garlic broth may do the trick for your cough, too, and it is easy to prepare. Smash 1 to 3 cloves garlic (depending on how strong you like your garlic), add 2 quarts water, and boil on low heat for one hour. Strain and sip slowly.

You can also chop up some garlic cloves and toss them into that pot of chicken soup.

GINGER. Ginger, which has antiviral properties, shares the limelight with licorice in this cough remedy.

HONEY. Honey has long been used in traditional Chinese medicine for coughs because it's a natural expectorant, promoting the flow of mucus. This is the simple recipe: Mix 1 tablespoon honey into 1 cup hot water and enjoy. Now how sweet is that? Squeeze some lemon juice in if you want a little tartness. Before bedtime, adults may add 1 tablespoon brandy or whiskey to aid in sleep.

LICORICE. If you love licorice, you're in for a treat with this remedy. Many folk remedies use licorice root to treat coughs and bronchial problems. It serves not only as a flavoring agent but also as a demulcent (a substance that soothes inflamed or irritated throats) and an expectorant. Real licorice or candy that's actually made with real licorice (look for licorice mass on the label) works best. Reach into your candy jar and slice up 1 ounce licorice sticks. Add 1 quart boiling water and steep for 24 hours. Drink throughout the day, adding a teaspoon of honey for sweetness.

MUSTARD SEED. An irritating but useful spice for wet coughs, mustard seed has sulfur-containing compounds that stimulate the flow of mucus. To get the full effect of the expectorant compounds, the mustard seeds must be broken and allowed to sit in water for 15 minutes. Crush 1 teaspoon mustard seeds or grind them in a coffee grinder. Place the seeds in a cup of warm water. Steep for 15 minutes. This concoction might be a little hard to swallow, so take it in $1/4$-cup doses throughout the day.

PEPPER. Pepper is a bit of an irritant (try sniffling some), but this characteristic is a plus for those suffering from coughs accompanied by thick mucus. The irritating property of pepper stimulates circulation and the flow of mucus in the airways and sinuses. Place 1 teaspoon black pepper into a cup and sweeten things up with the addition of 1 tablespoon honey. Fill with boiling water, steep for 10 to 15 minutes, stir, and sip.

THYME. Store-bought cough syrups are often so medicinal tasting that it's hard to get them down without gagging. Here's a sweet, herbal version, made of thyme, peppermint, mullein, licorice, and honey, that's guaranteed to go down the hatch easily. Thyme and peppermint help clear congested air passages and have antimicrobial and antispasmodic properties to relieve the hacking. Mullein and licorice soothe irritated membranes and help reduce inflammation.

To make the syrup, combine 2 teaspoons each dried thyme, peppermint, mullein, and licorice root into 1 cup boiling water. Cover and steep for half an hour. Strain and add $1/2$ cup honey. If the honey doesn't dissolve, heat the tea gently and stir. Store in the refrigerator in a covered container for up to three months. Take 1 teaspoon as needed.

* GINGER-LICORICE * (ANISE) TEA:

Combine 2 teaspoons freshly chopped gingerroot, 2 teaspoons aniseed, and if available, 1 teaspoon dried licorice root in 2 cups boiling water. Cover and steep for ten minutes. Strain and sweeten with 1 or 2 teaspoons honey. Drink $1/2$ cup every one to two hours, but no more than 3 cups a day.

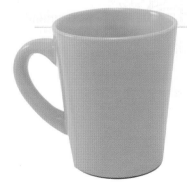

DEHYDRATION

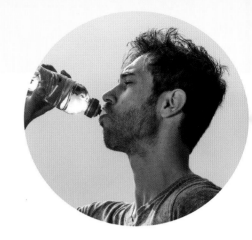

Every cell in your body needs water in order to function properly. In fact, an adult's body weight is 60 percent water while an infant's is up to 80 percent water. Other than oxygen, there's nothing that your body needs more than water. Water is so important because it has many critical -functions in the body. **Among other activities, water**

- Lubricates your joints and connective tissues

- Helps digest food

- Liquifies mucus when you've got a cold. This makes it easy to blow and cough it out.

- Eliminates body heat through sweat

- Carries oxygen, carbohydrates, and fats to working muscles, then carries away wastes such as carbon dioxide and lactic acid

- Flushes wastes from the body through urine

- Boosts endurance during prolonged exercise

- Dilutes and disperses medications and vitamins so they won't give you a bellyache

- Fights flight fatigue, often caused by dehydration from the dry air on the plane

- Wards off bladder infections by washing out harmful bacteria

- Helps curb your appetite

- Plumps up wrinkles. We have water in and around every cell in our bodies, and when water around those cells decreases, wrinkles happen.

- And yes, water quenches thirst. Thirst is our body's mechanism to alert us to insufficient fluids. If you're thirsty, it's time to restock.

THE GREAT ESCAPE

Each and every time you exhale, water escapes your body—up to as much as 2 cups per day. It evaporates invisibly from your skin—another 2 cups a day. And you urinate approximately $2\frac{1}{2}$ pints every 24 hours. Add it up, and you could be losing up to 10 cups of water every day, and that's before you break a sweat. By the time you feel thirsty, you've already lost one percent of your body's total water.

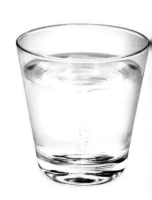

Because water has so many life-sustaining functions, dehydration isn't just a matter of being a little thirsty. The effects depend on the degree of dehydration, but a water shortage causes your kidneys to conserve water, which in turn can affect other body systems. You'll urinate less and can become constipated. As you become increasingly more dehydrated, these symptoms will develop:

- Diminished muscular endurance
- Dizziness
- Lack of energy
- Decreased concentration
- Drowsiness
- Irritability
- Headache
- Tachycardia (galloping heart rate)
- Increased body temperature
- Collapse
- Permanent organ damage or death

Older adults have a decreased sense of thirst, so they are even less able to tell when they need to drink than younger people. Indicators of dehydration in older adults include:

- Decreased urination
- Dry tongue
- Dry gums, or the inside cheeks are dry
- Mental confusion
- Upper-body weakness that's out of the ordinary
- Difficulty speaking
- Sunken eyes

HOW MUCH IS ENOUGH?

Obviously, you don't want to develop the problems listed above, so you have to ask: How much water do I need each day? Under normal conditions, the standard of 64 ounces a day is sufficient. That amount includes water from sources other than the tap. If you're an athlete or someone who spends a lot of time out in the sun sweating, you'll probably need more. A good way to tell if you're adequately hydrated is by observing the color of your urine. If it's dark yellow or amber, that's a sign that it's concentrated, meaning there's not enough water in the wastes that are being eliminated. If it's light, the color of lemon juice, that's normal.

Here are more facts about your urine:

- Some medications change the color, which means you can't keep an eye on your hydration level. Ask your physician about the medications you take, including over-the-counter drugs, vitamins, and minerals, that could change the color of your urine.

- Urine is normally darker and more concentrated in the morning, but with adequate hydration it lightens to lemon juice color and remains that way throughout the day.

- Bathroom breaks should happen every two to three hours. If you don't need to urinate for longer periods of time, you're not drinking enough water.

The simple cure for dehydration comes from the tap. Turn it on and drink. But there are other kitchen helpers that will keep you hydrated, too.

JET LAG * CURE

Some experts believe jet lag is caused by dehydration. But even if dehydration isn't the main cause of jet lag, it certainly is part of the jet-lag package. The air on board a plane is desert-dry, and you don't have access to fluids the way you do on land, unless you plan ahead. Those who are worried about making trips to the cramped airplane bathroom may consciously or subconsciously cut down on liquids.

If you're going to be traveling, here's how to avoid that jet lag:

- One hour before flying, drink a cup of ginger tea to soothe your nerves and provide last-minute hydration.

- On the plane, drink 2 to 3 cups water every couple of hours. Airlines may provide sufficient water, but to be sure you have a supply when you want it, take bottled water along. And skip the caffeinated drinks and alcohol. They are diuretics, which cause the body to lose water.

- After you arrive, don't stop hydrating. Be sure to continue drinking fluids.

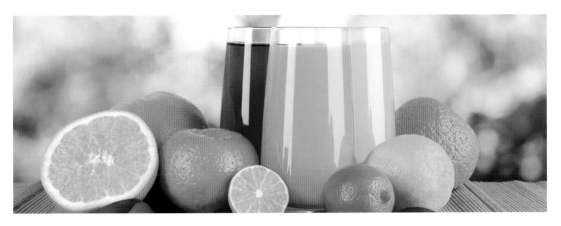

KITCHEN CURES

BANANAS. They have great water content and are especially good for restoring potassium that has vanished with dehydration.

BLAND FOODS. If you've experienced dehydration, stick to foods that are easily digested for the next 24 hours because stomach cramps are a symptom and can recur. Try soda crackers, rice, bananas, potatoes, and flavored gelatins. Gelatins are especially good since they are primarily made of water.

BOTTLED WATER. Easy to take along. Freeze some in the bottom of an empty bottle, then top if off with cold water when you're ready to go. You'll have cold water ready to drink for hours. If you know you'll need more than one bottle of cold water, grab another full bottle, drain about an inch from the top and freeze the whole thing. By the time the first bottle is empty, you'll have plenty of cold water in the second.

DECAFFEINATED TEA. Just another tasty way to get fluids in your body. Don't drink caffeinated tea, however, as caffeine is a mild diuretic.

FRUIT JUICE. It's liquid and has essential vitamins and minerals that need to be replenished.

ICE. Suck on it, or rub it on your body when you're overheated. This will help cool you down and prevent excess evaporation, which may lead to dehydration.

LIME JUICE. Add 1 teaspoon lime juice, a pinch of salt, and 1 teaspoon sugar to a pint of water. Sip the beverage throughout the day to cure mild dehydration.

RAISINS. They're packed with potassium, a body salt lost during dehydration.

POPSICLE. A great way to restore water to your body. It's an easy way to get fluids into kids, too.

SALT. If you're experiencing symptoms of mild dehydration or heat injury, or you're just plain sweating a lot, make sure you replace your salt. Don't just chug salt straight from the box, however. Try eating pretzels, salted crackers, or salty nuts.

SALTY FACTS

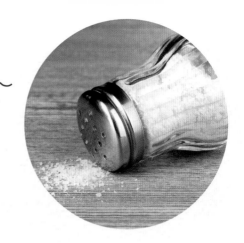

We always hear that we need to cut back on salt consumption, but salt hangs on to essential body water and is vital to these:

- Nerve impulse trans-mission

- Muscle contraction

- Heart muscle contraction

SPORTS DRINKS. Not only will they add water back into your system, they'll restore potassium and other essential electrolytes (a salt substance, such as potassium, sodium, and chlorine found in blood, tissue fluids, and cells that carry electrical impulses). For children, these adult drinks may be too harsh, so talk to your pharmacist about pediatric rehydration drinks now on the market.

WATERY FRUITS. Bananas are the number one fruit for rehydration, but watery fruits are a delicious and nutritious way to restore fluids. Try cantaloupe, watermelon, and strawberries. Watery vegetables such as cucumbers are good, too.

YOGURT. Or, cottage cheese. These have both sodium and potassium for replacing electrolytes.

MORE DO'S & DON'TS

- Don't cut back if you're retaining fluids. Water retention that's caused by salt needs to be addressed by increasing water consumption to flush salt from the body.

- Drink even when you're not thirsty. You're losing body fluids every second of the day, and they must be replaced.

- Don't depend on sport drinks or soft drinks for all your fluid requirements. They can come with side effects and calories. Plain old water is the best choice.

- Don't skip water if what comes from the tap tastes terrible. Bottled brands are available everywhere.

DENTAL DECAY

We take those choppers for granted, don't we? Except for that first year or two of life, they've always been there, ready to take on the grueling task of chewing. We douse them with sugar that erodes their enamel, require them to work overtime on foods hard enough to be called petrified, and then we forget the basics our parents taught us: Brush after every meal, and don't eat so many sweets.

Our teeth serve us well when they're in good order, but when something goes wrong, ouch! First comes that off-and-on-again little twinge, the one we ignore and hope will disappear. Next comes the sensitivity to hot and cold. And finally the full-out throb that hurts so bad that pulling the tooth out with a piece of string tied to a doorknob doesn't seem like such a bad way out.

Tooth problems hurt like a...toothache, and ultimately the solution comes in a dentist's chair, the drill screaming in your ear, your teeth clenching against the needle being jabbed right into your mouth.

Yes, we do abuse our teeth. And what's amazing about that is that overall, we're not neglecting our dental health. On average, 65 percent of all Americans visit their dentist regularly. So what's the deal? **Why the toothache?**

- Poor food choices
- Bacteria
- Bad brushing technique

- Not enough flossing
- Heredity
- Lack of professional care

Take your pick, the list is long. But there's also a kitchen list that can remedy some of your dental dilemmas.

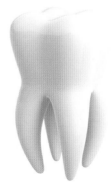

KITCHEN CURES

ALLSPICE. It helps relieve toothache. Wet your finger and dip it into the spice, then rub it along the gum line near the aching tooth. You can also steep some in a glass of warm water, then rinse your mouth with it. Not only does this rinse relieve pain, it also freshens your breath.

APPLES. Munching on a raw apple an hour after a meal cleans the teeth and helps heal the gums.

CARROTS. They're hard and crunchy, and like apples, they stimulate saliva production, which washes away food particles. Also, they have lots of beta-carotene, which may help prevent gum disease caused by dry mouth. Sweet potatoes, also loaded with beta-carotene, are another good choice.

CHEESE. You know that nasty bacteria that's just waiting to take a whack at your tooth enamel? Cheese is their sworn enemy. First, it stimulates the salivary glands to clean the mouth. According to studies, just a few ounces of hard cheese eaten after a meal may protect against decay. There's also evidence to suggest that fatty acids in cheese may have antibacterial properties. And finally, cheese proteins may actually coat and protect tooth enamel. So, here's another reason to "say cheese"!

CLOVES. Cloves contain eugenol, a chemical with natural antiseptic and anesthetic properties. That explains why ground cloves have been used to relieve toothaches for thousands of years. Moisten 1 teaspoon powdered cloves in olive oil and pack it into an aching cavity. Dentists still use a mixture of eugenol and zinc oxide before applying amalgam when filling teeth.

COCONUT OIL. Massage this into sore gums for relief.

CORIANDER. This spice, as well as thyme and green tea, has antibacterial properties. Brew a tea from your choice of the three and use as a mouth rinse after meals.

FIGS. To "strengthen" your teeth, eat 4 figs at one time, once a day. Chew well and slowly. This stimulates the saliva flow and cleanses the mouth.

LEMON JUICE. Squeeze the juice of half a lemon into a cup full of water and drink to staunch bleeding gums and gingivitis. Don't take lemon juice full strength, as it can erode tooth enamel.

MELON. Any melon will do. One hour after eating, chew some melon slowly. It will help stop gums from bleeding.

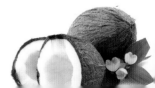

MILK. Milk is alkaline, which doesn't erode tooth enamel like acidic fruit juices and soft drinks do. It's also calcium-rich, which is vital for strong teeth and bones. Check your fridge for these other calcium-packed foods while you're there: yogurt, broccoli, Swiss chard, and salmon.

ORANGE JUICE. Add ½ teaspoon natural sugar and a pinch of cumin to 1 cup fresh orange juice to help bleeding gums. Rinse with water afterward.

SAGE. Add 2 teaspoons sage to 2 cups water, then boil. Cool for 15 minutes, then swish in your mouth for several minutes. Sage has an antibacterial property that may reduce decay.

SALSA. The spicier the better. Foods that make your mouth water actually fight dental decay. They stimulate the salivary glands, and all the extra saliva cleans your teeth and gums. And if that salsa is too hot, the water you'll drink to cool the burn will clean your mouth, too.

SESAME SEEDS. Chew a handful slowly but don't swallow. Brush your teeth with a dry toothbrush, using the chewed seeds as you would a toothpaste. They will both clean and polish.

SESAME OIL. Gargling with warm sesame oil is an Ayurvedic treatment for gum disease. Take a mouthful and swish it around twice a day, then rinse. It's also said that this simple gargle can reduce cheek wrinkles. What a great bonus!

STRAWBERRIES. They're a wonderful tooth whitener. Rub the juice on the teeth and leave for five minutes. Then rinse off with warm water that has a pinch of baking soda dissolved in it.

TEA BAG. Black tea contains fluoride that can suppress the growth of bacteria that cause decay and dental plaque, the sticky white film that forms on your teeth. (When it hardens, it's called tartar.) Drop a tea bag of black tea into a cup of hot water, and let it brew for six minutes. This will allow the maximum amount of fluoride to escape into the water. Squeeze the tea bag into the water before discarding it to get that last little bit of fluoride. Use the tea as a rinse to prevent plaque buildup after you eat sweets.

VINEGAR. Here's an easy but temporary toothache fix. Try rinsing your mouth with a mixture of 4 ounces warm water, 2 tablespoons vinegar, and 1 tablespoon salt.

WATERCRESS. Chew fresh watercress vseveral times a day to treat sore or bleeding gums.

ENAMEL BUSTERS

Fruits containing citric acid, such as oranges and grapefruit, can erode the enamel in teeth, so eat them only with meals. If you do eat them as a snack or drink fresh citrus fruit juice, swish your mouth out with water afterward. Do the same when you drink colas and other carbonated beverages.

* FROZEN FRUIT-JUICE FIASCO

We all love these treats, especially in the summer when it's hot and they're so refreshing. And they seem like such a healthy treat, too. But these chilly goodies are rotting your teeth.

How? The acid content in these juice bars is so high that the normally protective saliva fails to clean your teeth. To make matters worse, you suck on the bars or hold them in your mouth until they melt, prolonging the acidic exposure. Definitely not tooth friendly. So after you eat the treat, swish with some water.

DENTURE DISCOMFORT

Anyone who has donned a set of dentures knows discomfort is part of the process. There are two periods when discomfort is at its peak: the initial days of wearing the new device and several years later when the dentures may not fit properly.

The cause of the discomfort isn't a mystery. After the teeth are extracted, the dentures sit on the bony ridge that's leftover. Without the stability of permanent teeth, this bony ridge changes and shrinks over the years while the dentures remained fixed. Slipping and sliding dentures cause sore spots, which is the reason for much of denture discomfort. Dentures may not fit like a glove, but you shouldn't suffer. There are a variety of ways to prevent and resolve denture discomfort.

KITCHEN CURES

ANISEED. This gentle herbal mouth rinse is perfect for sensitive mouths. Combine 2 teaspoons crushed aniseed, 1 tablespoon peppermint leaves, and 2 cups boiling water. Cover and steep for eight hours. Strain and add 1 teaspoon myrrh tincture, which acts as an antiseptic and preservative. Use 2 tablespoons twice a day for rinsing. The remainder of the rinse can be stored in a glass bottle. Shake before using.

CLOVE. The clove has been used as a remedy for aching mouths since antiquity. The clove remedy started in Asian folk medicine, and the concept traveled along trade routes to Europe and the Mediterranean along with the spice itself. By the third century B.C. the clove was the universal folk remedy for mouth and dental pain in the Mediterranean. Clove's medicinal use continued into the nineteenth century, when dentists used clove oil to relieve dental pain. Even today dentists use eugenol, a major ingredient in clove oil, as a pain reliever and to disinfect dental abscesses. Perhaps cloves' timeless popularity stems from the fact that they not only eliminate pain but also smell terrific. There's nothing like having a fresh and pain-free mouth all in one. To tap into these healing properties, blend 1 teaspoon cloves into a powder using a coffee grinder or use $1/2$ teaspoon prepackaged ground cloves. Moisten with olive oil and dab around a mouth or gum sore.

FIGS. Figs are fabulous for fighting mouth sores. The fig remedy, however, requires some time, coordination, and of course, a fresh fig. Once you locate the prized fruit, cut it in half and set one half between your cheek and the sore spot on your gum. The open side of the fig should touch the gum. This is a bit tricky to keep in place, so plan on watching TV or keeping still while you fig out.

SOFT FOODS. Eat like a baby during the adjustment period. You don't have to mash peas in a blender, but you should stick to soft, easy-to-chew foods such as soups, stews, and pastas (macaroni and cheese). If you chew on hard foods, such as carrots and pretzels, you'll risk damaging tender gum tissues that are still reeling from the shock of losing their natural teeth. For dessert, enjoy puddings, gelatin, and applesauce.

SALT. Gargling with warm salt water may help denture wearers breeze through the adjustment phase sans mouth sores. Prevent sore spots from becoming infected or inflamed by rinsing every three to four hours. The salt water cleans out bacteria, shrinks swollen tissue, and helps toughen the tender tissue. Make a saltwater rinse by adding $\frac{1}{2}$ teaspoon salt to 4 ounces warm water. Gargle and spit. Do this twice daily.

AFTER THE MEAL

After teeth are extracted and new dentures fit, it's of prime importance to keep your new choppers sparkling clean. Excess bacteria buildup on dentures can retard the gum's healing process. Plain old soap, warm water, and a hand brush do a grand job at cleaning. Scrub at least twice a day and rinse well.

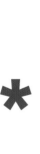

DEPRESSION

There are many times in the course of life that you may feel overwhelmed and distraught.

If you didn't feel like singing the blues now and again you wouldn't be human. It's actually very healthy to get down from time to time. It's when that down-in-the-dumps feeling begins to stick around longer than a couple of weeks that you might be suffering from a more serious condition, such as clinical depression. If you are experiencing a bout of depression, don't feel alone. Mental health experts say at least 30 million people deal with mild depression every year, and 18.8 million Americans are diagnosed with a more serious form of depression annually.

MAJOR OR MINOR?

Though it'd be nice to go through life pretending like you're in a Brady Bunch episode, it's not realistic. There are going to be times when life throws you a few curveballs. Perhaps you suddenly lose a parent or your spouse is diagnosed with a major illness. Feeling depressed during tough times is normal. Mild depression is something everyone encounters. But sometimes stressful situations can cause more than a few days of sadness.

If your hopeless feelings begin to become more intense and last more than a couple of weeks, you could be experiencing clinical depression. Major depression, one form of clinical depression, may only happen once in your lifetime, or it may come back several times. Major depression usually lasts weeks or months and is disabling. It can cause you to lose interest in work, sleep, eating, or going out to dinner with a friend. A less severe form of clinical depression is dysthymia.

Dysthymia isn't as emotionally crippling as major depression. With dysthymia you go about your life, attending soccer games and birthday parties, but it feels as though there's a gray cloud hanging over your life. Dysthymia is a chronic condition. And people with dysthymia may suffer bouts of major depression throughout their lives.

CAUSES OF DEPRESSION

Researchers have discovered that depression can run in the family. That doesn't mean that you'll definitely suffer bouts of depression if your mother or father did. But if you encounter a stressful situation, such as losing your job, you'll be more likely to slip into a major depression than someone who doesn't have a genetic link to the condition

Physiologically most types of depression are related to a malfunction in neurotransmitters in the brain. Researchers have discovered that if there is a glitch in the way neurotransmitters communicate, you can experience problems with mood, sleeping, and eating. Also, people who are more susceptible to depression physiologically tend to overreact to stress. **Other causes of depression include:**

- Major stresses, such as going through a serious illness or losing someone close to you.

- Hormonal changes. As hormones fluctuate—after having a baby, before and during menstruation, and during menopause—women tend to suffer more depression.

- Medications. Check with your doctor if you've recently started a new medication and are feeling symptoms of depression.

KITCHEN CURES

BRAZIL NUTS. Selenium, a trace mineral found abundantly in Brazil nuts (100 mcg in one nut), can help ease depression. Studies have shown that people who had low levels of selenium tended to be more anxious, depressed, and tired. Once they ate foods containing selenium, however, they felt better. Other selenium-rich foods are tuna, swordfish, oysters, and sunflower seeds.

CHICKEN. Low levels of vitamin B6 may be an instigator of depression, especially in women on birth control pills. Vitamin B6 is necessary for the body to make serotonin, a neurotransmitter. The RDA for vitamin B6 is 1.3 mg for men and women up to age 50; after age 50 the amount increases to 1.7 mg for men and 1.5 mg for women. Pregnant and nursing mothers need more. There are 0.5 mg of vitamin B6 in 3 ounces of chicken.

TOP 10 CAUSES OF STRESS

The more stress you have in your life, the more likely you will experience depression. That's especially true of the following life events:

Death of a spouse
Divorce
Menopause
Separation from living partner
Death of close family member
Loss of job
Seriously personal injury or illness
Marriage
Retirement
Illness of family member

COFFEE. If you're a regular morning coffee drinker, you know what life can be like if you don't have your morning cup. You get a headache, you're cranky, and you feel bad. Well, researchers are finding that caffeine can indeed alter your mood. It makes you less irritable and helps you feel better. Experts do think that having a cup or two of coffee a day may indeed help ease mild depression. But don't go overboard. Downing too much caffeine can make you jittery and may even make you more anxious.

GARLIC. German researchers studying garlic's effect on cholesterol discovered that participants being treated with garlic experience an elevation in mood. So try a little garlic therapy if you're feeling down.

SPINACH. Studies are finding that a folic acid deficiency is a major cause of depression. Scientists began to suspect a link between this B vitamin and the brain when they discovered that people diagnosed with depression have lower levels of folic acid than the general population. It seems that folic acid deficiency causes serotonin levels to fall, which can lead to feelings of depression. Ironically enough, folic acid deficiency is one of the most common nutrient deficiencies in women. But the good news is you only need about 200 mcg a day to meet your folic acid needs. That adds up to about ¾ cup of cooked spinach.

TUNA. The brain is one of the richest sources of fatty acids in the body. And research is finding that depressed people have lower levels of omega-3 fatty acids. This polyunsaturated fat is found mostly in fatty fish. Researchers believe that getting enough omega-3 fatty acids is essential to ensure the brain is at its healthiest. And a healthy brain is less likely to become seriously depressed.

✳ FOODS TO AVOID

If you're dealing with mild depression, there are some practical things you can do to lift your mood.

- Junk the junk food. Sure that sugar high feels good, but when you go through detox a couple of hours after that cupcake, you can feel terrible. Try skipping the sugary stuff and eating something more nutritious.

- Abstain from alcohol. Alcohol is known to aggravate a depressed mood.

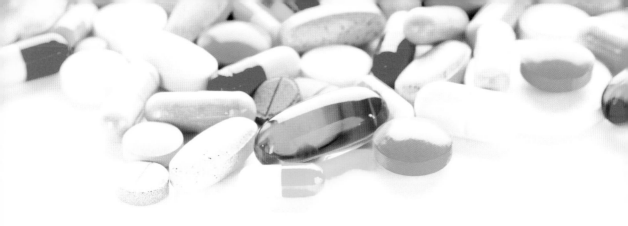

EAT TO LIVE, HAPPILY

What you eat affects how you feel, but what you don't eat may do the same. Depression has been linked to low levels of many nutrients, such as biotin, calcium, copper, iron, magnesium, pantothenic acid, potassium, pyridoxine, riboflavin, thiamin, vitamin C, vitamin E, and zinc. So if you are dealing with a mild depression, take a look at what you're eating. Some changes in your diet may make a difference in your mood.

Biotin (B7): Eggs, almonds, avocados, cauliflower

Calcium: Milk, yogurt, cheese, kale, broccoli

Copper: Shellfish, especially oysters, nuts, baked potatoes, legumes

Iron: Beans and lentils, tofu, baked potatoes, spinach, broccoli, beef, poultry

Magnesium: Whole grains, spinach, edamame, dark leafy greens, quinoa

Pantothenic acid (B5): Fortified breakfast cereals, beef liver, shiitake mushrooms, sunflower seeds, chicken, tuna, avocados

Potassium: Apricots, lentils, prunes, squash, raisins, baked potatoes, kidney beans

Pyridoxine (B6): Along with chicken, mentioned above, chickpeas, boiled potatoes, salmon, beef liver, and tuna

Riboflavin (B2): Beef liver, fortified breakfast cereals, oats, yogurt, milk, clams, portabella mushrooms

Thiamin (B1): Fortified breakfast cereals, rice, trout, black beans, mussels

Vitamin C: Red and green peppers, oranges and orange juice, grapefruit, kiwi, broccoli, strawberries

Vitamin E: Sunflower seeds, almonds, sunflower and safflower oil, hazelnuts, peanuts and peanut oil

Zinc: Oysters (three ounces of oysters have 493 percent of the recommended daily allowance), beef, crab and lobster, fortified breakfast cereals

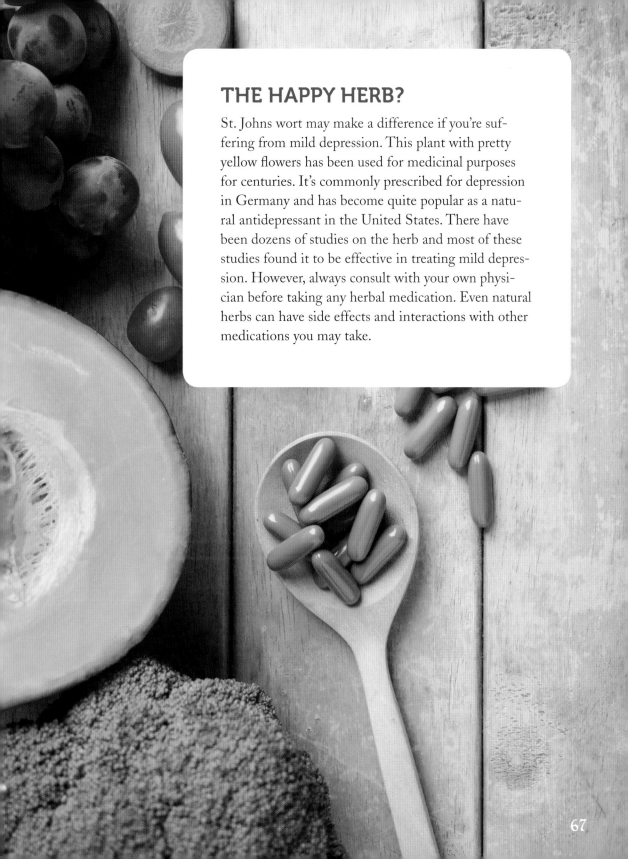

THE HAPPY HERB?

St. Johns wort may make a difference if you're suffering from mild depression. This plant with pretty yellow flowers has been used for medicinal purposes for centuries. It's commonly prescribed for depression in Germany and has become quite popular as a natural antidepressant in the United States. There have been dozens of studies on the herb and most of these studies found it to be effective in treating mild depression. However, always consult with your own physician before taking any herbal medication. Even natural herbs can have side effects and interactions with other medications you may take.

DIABETES

Diabetes is a disease that reduces, or stops, the body's ability to produce or respond to insulin, a hormone produced in the pancreas. Insulin's role is to open the door for glucose, a form of sugar, to enter the body's cells so that it can be used for energy. When the body has a problem metabolizing glucose, it builds up in the blood, and the body's cells starve.

THERE ARE TWO MAJOR TYPES OF DIABETES:

Type 1. The body produces no insulin at all, and daily insulin shots are required. This disease used to be called juvenile diabetes because there is a higher rate of diagnosis among children ages 10 to 14. It is also referred to as insulin-dependent diabetes because injections of insulin are required to control blood glucose. The cause isn't known, but Type 1 tends to run in families. A much smaller number of people with diabetes have Type 1—only five percent.

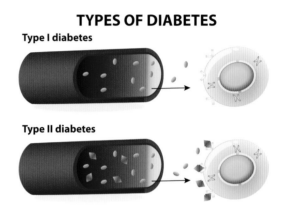

TYPES OF DIABETES

Type I diabetes

Type II diabetes

Type 2. This is the most common form of diabetes, and it occurs when the body is insulin resistant. That could be either because the body fails to make enough insulin or because it doesn't properly use the insulin it does produce. The cause is often poor dietary habits, sedentary lifestyle, and obesity. Those with Type 2 may or may not need oral medication or insulin, depending on how their body responds to changes in diet and exercise.

Here's the risk list for diabetes. Do any of these describe you?

- Over age 45
- Family history of diabetes
- Overweight
- Don't exercise regularly
- Low HDL cholesterol or high triglycerides
- Member of an at-risk ethnic group

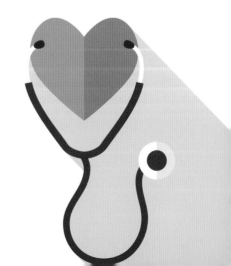

SYMPTOMS

In children, the symptoms of the onset of Type 1 diabetes may be similar to flu symptoms. **They also may include these:**

- Frequent urination
- Unusual thirst
- Extreme hunger

- Unexplained weight loss
- Extreme fatigue
- Irritability

Symptoms of Type 2 diabetes include:

- Any of the Type 1 symptoms
- Frequent infections, including those of the skin, gums, and bladder
- Blurred vision

- Sores that are slow to heal
- Tingling or numbness in hands or feet
- In women, recurring vaginitis

TREATMENT

There is no cure for diabetes, but it can be controlled. And control is essential because diabetes can lead to heart disease, stroke, kidney disease and failure, blindness, and amputation if not treated. This profile will not address diabetic medical treatment, including prescribed diabetic diets. Those specifics must be left up to your physician and dietitian. But this profile will cover the go-alongs; things from your kitchen that can make the diabetic experience easier. Note, however, that nothing contained in this profile is intended to stop or replace your prescribed diabetic care!

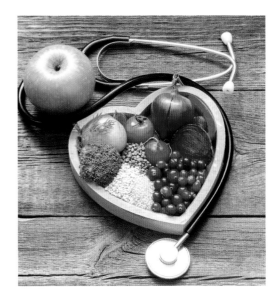

Diabetes is a complex disease, affecting many parts of the body. Some of the problems of the disease can be relieved with simple things right from the kitchen, though. And for a person with diabetes, a little relief never hurts.

KITCHEN CURES

ASPARAGUS. This vegetable is a mild diuretic that's said to be beneficial in the control of diabetes. Eat it steamed and drizzled with olive oil and lemon juice.

BEANS. They've been known to reduce blood sugar in some people. Kidney beans are the best, fresh in the pod. Boil 2 ounces of sliced pods in 4 quarts of water. Simmer four hours. Strain and cool the liquid for eight hours. Strain again. Drink 1 glassful every two hours. In the absence of kidney bean pods, fresh green beans will work, too. Beans eaten with a meal, just as they are, have been known to lessen the rise in blood sugar that comes after the meal.

GARLIC. Eating a combination of garlic, parsley, and watercress may shave a few points off the blood sugar. Try combining these herbs in a vegetable stir-fry or salad.

LEMON. A tasty substitute for salt. It's great squeezed into a diet cola, too. It cuts the aftertaste.

OLIVE OIL. Studies indicate this may reduce blood sugar levels. Use it in salad dressing or wherever cooking oils are indicated. For an inexpensive and easy no-stick olive oil spray-on coating, buy an oil mister in any department store kitchen supply area and use it to spray your pans before cooking.

PARSLEY. Steep into a tea and drink. This may act as a diuretic as well as lower blood sugar.

PEANUT BUTTER. After you've experienced an episode of low blood sugar and corrected it, follow up with a protein and carbohydrate snack. Peanut butter on a couple of crackers supplies both, and it's easy to fix when you may still feel a little jittery. Just avoid brands that contain added sugar, glucose, or jelly.

SALT SHAKER. Set it aside, put it back in the cupboard, hide it. High blood pressure is a side effect of diabetes, and that salt's a no-no. So don't cook with it, and don't make it handy to grab when you eat a meal or snack. If it's out of sight, or inconvenient to get, you might just skip it. Instead, reach for a nice herb or spice blend that's sodium free. Make one yourself with your favorite spices or buy one at the store.

SUGAR. Yes, even people with diabetes need it occasionally, when their blood sugar goes too low. A spoonful of straight sugar will work, as will a piece of hard candy. Just be sure it's not sugarless.

WATERCRESS. This is said to strengthen the natural defense systems of people who have diabetes. It's also a mild diuretic. Wash the leaves thoroughly, and add them to a salad. Or smear a little cream cheese on a slice of bread, then top with watercress for a delicious open-faced sandwich.

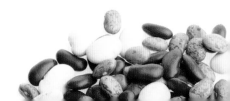

MORE DO'S AND DON'TS

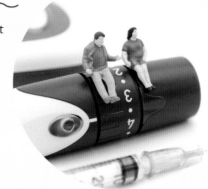

- Use a fork to apply salad dressing and sauces to limit your intake of sugar, as well as fat and cholesterol. Instead of dumping the dressing or sauce all over your food, have it served "on the side" and dip your fork into it, then pick up your food. You'll get the flavor without all the extra goop.

- Use a notebook to keep track of glucose readings, medication schedules, and symptoms.

- Monitor your glucose levels regularly via finger sticks. That's the only way you can accurately gauge how you're doing. Record the results for your doctor and dietician.

- Maintain a regular eating schedule. Your body needs it.

- Eat foods with a low glycemic index, as they release sugar slowly into the bloodstream.

- If your blood sugar level drops to the point that you need a quick pick-me-up, candy's fine, but skip the chocolate. Its high fat content slows the absorption of sugar, so it doesn't work quickly enough.

- As fruits are dehydrated, the sugar in them becomes concentrated. Limit your intake of dried fruit to two or three times a week or less.

FISHY FACT

According to a Dutch study, fish eaters are half as likely to get Type 2 diabetes as people who don't eat fish. The amount consumed was small—1 ounce a day. Most likely the omega-3 oil found in fish helps the pancreas handle glucose.

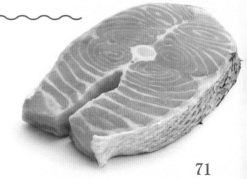

71

DIARRHEA

It's got all kinds of colorful nicknames, including "Greased Lightning," "Turkey Trots," and "Montezuma's Revenge." You may have even heard your 11-year-old singing a catchy little ditty about it. But just saying the word diarrhea gets a reaction from most people—they either giggle or turn pale. Diarrhea is probably one of the most unpleasant problems that plagues us. And it's a common malady. Americans usually suffer from diarrhea a couple times a year. For most adults, diarrhea isn't serious. And it does give you a chance to ponder some redecorating ideas for the bathroom.

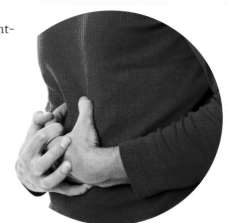

THE RUNDOWN ON DIARRHEA

On a typical day, you eat a hoagie and drink an iced tea and your meal makes its way through the digestive system without any problems. By the time it reaches the intestines, your food is mostly fluid with bits of solid material. The intestines reabsorb most of the fluid, and the solid stuff is excreted in the usual fashion. But when you've got diarrhea, something blocks the intestine's ability to absorb fluid. You've got loads of watery fluids mixed in with your stool, and you get that "gotta go" feeling.

There are essentially two types of diarrhea: acute and chronic. Thankfully, the vast majority of diarrhea is acute, or short term. This type of diarrhea keeps you on the toilet for a couple of days but doesn't stick around long. Acute diarrhea is also known as non-inflammatory diarrhea. Its symptoms are what most people associate with the condition: watery, frequent stools accompanied by stomach cramps, gas, and nausea.

Acute diarrhea usually has a bacterial or viral culprit. Gastroenteritis, mistakenly called the "stomach flu," is one of the most common infections that cause diarrhea. Gastroenteritis can be caused by many different viruses. Eating or drinking foods contaminated with bacteria can also cause diarrhea. Other causes of acute diarrhea are lactose intolerance, sweeteners such as sorbitol, over-the-counter antacids that contain magnesium, too much vitamin C, and some antibiotics.

If you have chronic, or long-term, diarrhea that comes on suddenly and stays for weeks, you may have a more serious condition such as irritable bowel syndrome or a severe food allergy.

DEHYDRATION DANGERS

With any kind of diarrhea you lose a lot of fluids. One of the quickest ways you can end up going from the bathroom to the emergency room is to take a pass on liquids while you're sick. Fluids not only keep things running smoothly in your body, they also keep electrolyte levels balanced. Electrolytes are sodium, potassium, and chloride salts that your body needs for proper organ function. An electrolyte imbalance can cause your heart to beat irregularly, causing life-threatening problems. Though drinking or eating anything while you're running back and forth to the bathroom might sound grotesque, it will help make you more comfortable and get you back on your feet more quickly.

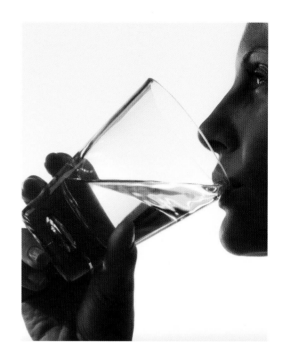

Though experts don't see eye to eye on what fluids are best during a bout with diarrhea, they do agree that getting two to three quarts of fluid a day is a good idea. When you drink, it's easier on the tummy if you sip instead of gulp (who has the energy for gulping?) and if you drink cool, not cold or hot, fluids. Here are some tried-and-true fluids that should get you through the rough days.

- Decaffeinated tea with a little sugar
- Sports drinks
- Commercially available electrolyte replacement drinks for children
- Bouillon
- Chicken broth
- Orange juice

Though it may not sound logical to put diarrhea and food in the same sentence, if you don't put something in your body while you're enduring tummy troubles, you might end up getting sicker. There are loads of good things from the kitchen that will ease your grumbling stomach, and there are a few things that will prevent those diarrhea-causing agents from coming back for a return engagement.

KITCHEN CURES

BANANA. Long known as a soother for tummy trouble, this potassium-rich fruit can restore nutrients and is easy to digest.

BLUEBERRIES. Blueberry root is a long-time folk remedy for diarrhea. In Sweden, doctors prescribe a soup made with dried blueberries for tummy problems. Blueberries are rich in anthocyanosides, which have antioxidant and antibacterial properties, as well as tannins, which combat diarrhea.

CHAMOMILE TEA. Chamomile is good for treating intestinal inflammation, and it has antispasmodic properties as well. You can brew yourself a cup of chamomile tea from packaged tea bags, or you can buy chamomile flowers and steep 1 teaspoon of them and 1 teaspoon of peppermint leaves in a cup of boiling water for fifteen minutes. Drink 3 cups a day.

COOKED CEREALS. Starchy foods, such as precooked rice or tapioca cereals, can help ease your tummy. Prepare the cereal according to the directions on the box, making it as thick as you can stomach it. Just avoid adding too much sugar or salt, as these can aggravate diarrhea. It's probably a good idea to avoid oatmeal since it's high in fiber and your intestines can't tolerate the added bulk during a bout with diarrhea.

FENUGREEK SEEDS. Science has given the nod to this folk remedy. But this one is for adults only. Mix $1/2$ teaspoon fenugreek seeds with water and drink up.

ORANGE PEEL. Orange peel tea is a folk remedy that is believed to aid in digestion. Place a chopped orange peel (preferably from an organic orange, as peels otherwise may contain pesticides and dyes) into a pot and cover with 1 pint boiling water. Let it stand until the water is cooled. You can sweeten it with sugar or honey.

POTATOES. This is another starchy food that can help restore nutrients and comfort your stomach. But eating french fries won't help. Fried foods tend to aggravate an aching tummy. Other root vegetables such as carrots (cooked, of course) are also easy on an upset stomach, and they are loaded with nutrients.

RICE. Cooked white rice is another starchy food that can be handled by someone recovering from diarrhea.

SUGAR. Mix 4 teaspoons sugar and $1/2$ teaspoon salt with 1 quart water. Mixing electrolytes (such as salt) with a form of glucose (sugar) helps the body to better absorb the nutrients.

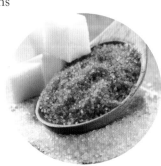

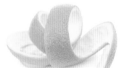

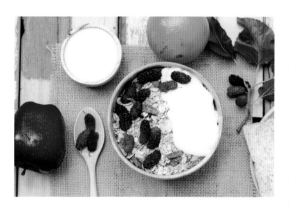

YOGURT. Look for yogurt with live cultures. These "cultures" are friendly bacteria that can go in and line your intestines, providing you protection from the bad guys. If you've already got diarrhea, yogurt can help produce lactic acid in your intestines, which can kill off the nasty bacteria and get you feeling better, faster.

NO MORE EXCUSES TO BE A BRAT

Although the classic BRAT (bananas, rice, applesauce, and toast) diet is touted as the best for refeeding after a bout with diarrhea, The American Academy of Pediatrics considers that diet too low in energy density, protein, and fat for children. While those foods can be tolerated, the Academy suggests introducing complex carbohydrates (rice, wheat, potatoes, bread, and cereals), lean meats, yogurt, fruits, and vegetables. Research shows these foods, too, are well-tolerated. Foods to avoid giving your children include those that are high in fat, salt, or sugar (including juice and soft drinks).

✳ MILK'S NOT
ALWAYS GOOD
✳ FOR YOU

Between 70 and 90 percent of Asian, African-American, Native American, and Mediterranean adults lack the enzyme lactase, which is responsible for digesting lactose, a sugar found in milk. Lactose intolerance is the most common reason for chronic diarrhea.

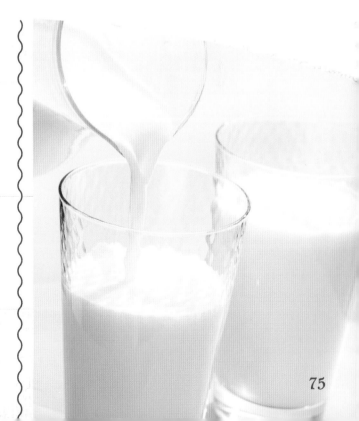

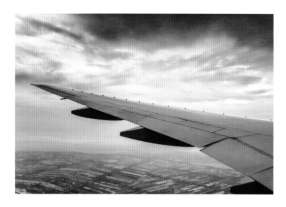

AVOIDING TRAVELER'S DIARRHEA

The announcer said, "Congratulations, you've just won a five-day, four-night stay at a posh resort in the tropical paradise of your choice." Unfortunately, he didn't mention that paradise came with a bevy of food-borne parasites. Forty to sixty percent of Americans who travel abroad will end up with a case of traveler's diarrhea, usually within four to six days of arrival in a foreign country. It's most often caused by a bacteria, such as *E. coli*, that wanders into the intestines and beds down. Once you've got it, it can take hold with a vengeance and last for weeks.

You can avoid getting traveler's diarrhea by avoiding the bacteria that cause it. The best way to do that is to read up on potential bacterial invasions in your country of choice—see the Centers for Disease Control Web site www.cdc.gov to get a lowdown on your destination. And take these practical precautions to avoid any of Montezuma's gifts.

- **Make sure raw foods are cooked or boiled.** Don't eat anything that appears rare. If you are eating fruit, make sure it has a peel.

- **Take care of your own stuff.** Peel your own fruit. Open your own bottle of water. The fruit on the buffet table may have been washed in contaminated water. That open bottle of water could be from the tap.

- **Go back on the bottle.** Drink only bottled water, preferably the bubbly kind. Carbonation seems to kill some bacteria. If you can't get bottled water, invest in a portable water filter.

- **Don't drink the water.** Don't drink tap water in any form—spritzed over vegetables, in the form of ice cubes, in a pitcher of lemonade, etc.

- **Eat it hot.** Only eat food that is hot to the touch, and eat as quickly as you can. Food that has cooled is a prime spot for nasty bacteria.

- If you do get diarrhea and aren't careful to replace the fluid you're losing, you might be in danger of dehydrating. There are certain age-groups, such as children and the elderly, who are more in danger of dehydrating, and special care needs to be taken when they have diarrhea.

✳ FOODS to AVOID ～～～

- **Caffeine.** It stimulates the nervous system, including the intestines.

- **Sweeteners such as sorbitol, xylitol, and mannitol.** These are mostly found in fruit juices, such as apple juice, and sugarless candy.

- **Milk and cheese.** The intestines work extra hard to digest the enzymes in these dairy products. While your body is down for the count, and even a few days after you're better, you might want to avoid dairy of any kind except for yogurt.

- **Fiber.** Now is not the time to bulk up. Fiber is simply too hard for an aching tummy to digest.

- **Sugar.** Some sugar is good during a case of diarrhea—it can help you absorb electrolytes needed for rehydration—but too much can make things worse.

DIVERTICULAR DISEASE

Diverticulosis is a common condition in which small pouches, called diverticula, develop in the colon. It happens when the inner lining of the large intestine is forced, under pressure, through weak spots in the outer layer of the colon. No one is sure what causes diverticulosis, but a low-fiber diet and lack of exercise have been shown to put you at greater risk. The diverticular pouches are present in about 50 percent of people over age 60, and they themselves are not much of a problem. However, when a food particle or piece of waste material lodges in the pouches, it can become inflamed and cause a more serious illness called diverticulitis. Diverticulitis can range from a mild infection to a severe one requiring hospitalization and even surgery.

SYMPTOMS

Diverticulosis usually causes no symptoms. Most people won't even know they have the condition unless it has shown up on a routine colonoscopy or developed into diverticulitis. But diverticulitis does have symptoms, including

- Abdominal cramping, usually more severe on the lower-left side
- Abdominal pain triggered by touch
- Nausea
- Gas, belching, bloating

- Fever
- Diarrhea, constipation, or very thin stools
- Blood in the stools
- General feeling of being tired or run-down

If you have any of these symptoms, don't self-diagnose. Call a doctor or, if the symptoms are severe, get yourself to the doctor's office or an emergency room. Diverticulitis that's untreated can lead to perforation of the colon, formation of an abscess, or peritonitis, a life-threatening infection of the lining of the abdominal cavity.

Diverticula don't go away. Once you have them, you're stuck with them. It's a good idea to adjust your lifestyle to avoid flare-ups, and for mild symptoms there's relief to be found in the kitchen.

Warning! The following are to help prevent the development of diverticulitis or to ease the mildest of symptoms. For all other symptoms, see a doctor!

KITCHEN CURES

BARLEY. This grain is a digestive anti-inflammatory. Add some to vegetable soup or stew. Or buy some barley flour, flakes, and grits.

BROWN RICE. It's easy on the digestive system, rich in fiber, and calms inflammation and spasms in the colon. Eat it plain or as a dessert with a little honey, mix it with vegetables for a stir-fry, try it in the morning as a breakfast food instead of oatmeal, or boil it for a tea and drink the liquid in addition to eating the rice. There are no limits to the ways you can serve up brown rice.

GARLIC. This can help prevent infection. Eat 1 clove, three times a day. Chop it into a salad or add it to soup or stew. Pasta sauce, however, is not a good choice since tomato-based, spicy, and acidic foods can exacerbate symptoms.

PAPAYA. This soothes diverticulitis. Find a nice, ripe, red-tinged papaya, cut it open, toss away the seeds, and eat. Use it in a fruit salad; it's especially good with melons. Or put it in the blender and make juice. Add a little honey to sweeten it up, if necessary. Papaya has an unusual but enjoyable flavor.

PEAR. Another fruit that can soothe inflammation, pears don't need any doctoring to eat. Simply find one that's ripe and enjoy.

POTATOES. They're tasty and nourishing, and they have soothing, anti-inflammatory properties that are especially good for digestive woes. Because grease can aggravate diverticulitis, avoid fried potatoes of any sort. But any other cooking method will do: baking, broiling, or boiling.

FABULOUS FIBER (A.K.A. BULK)

Fiber, also known as bulk, is essential to alleviating problems associated with diverticulitis and for having a healthy colon. Everyone needs 25 to 30 grams a day. The problem is, even though we think we're getting plenty of fiber, most of us are getting only half of what we need.

Remember, though, to add fiber to your diet slowly at first. Try a little one day, skip a day, then add a little more the next. Too much too soon can lead to constipation. And be sure to

FOODS TO SKIP

- Skip the caffeine. It can cause digestive upset.

- Cut back on red meats. They weaken the wall of the colon, which is where the pouches in diverticulosis start.

drink plenty of water as you're adding fiber—at least 8 glasses a day. That helps push all that added fiber on through the digestive system. The faster it's gone, the less likely the chances of it, or any other foods, getting lodged in one of the diverticula and causing a problem.

HERBAL CURES

There are a variety of herbs that can help soothe your digestive tract. Try these:

Chamomile. This is a mild pain reliever, and it has properties that smooth digestion. Drink it as a tea or use the essential oil, mixed with lavender oil, to massage the abdomen, especially over the lower-left area when it's tender. Add it to bathwater, too.

Dandelion. That backyard weed has anti-inflammatory properties that work well in the digestive tract. Dandelions can be eaten in a variety of ways:

- Steep fresh tender leaves for a tea.

- Scrub and steam the root and add it to steamed, mixed vegetables.

- Make a salad by tossing 2 cups mixed lettuce leaves with $1/2$ cup dandelion greens. Add 3 tablespoons olive oil and the juice of $1/2$ lemon. Toss well. If you pick your own dandelion leaves, just be sure you harvest them from an area that is free of pesticides and fertilizers and away from roadways.

Teas. Any of these can be used as tea that can relieve the symptoms of diverticulitis: fenugreek seed, marshmallow root, slippery-elm bark. If you don't have them on hand, try the health food store.

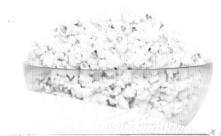

TRUE OR NOT?

One of the traditional warnings that used to come with a diagnosis of diverticulosis was to avoid nuts, popcorn, and seeds. Why? Because they can lodge in the diverticula and cause inflammation. The truth is, some doctors still say to avoid these, but there's no evidence that these foods cause diverticulitis, according to the National Institutes of Health. What should you do? Listen to your gut. If you love popcorn, for example, try a small amount and see what happens. If it causes problems, don't eat it again. If it doesn't, enjoy it in moderation. Just be sure to chew those seeds and nuts well. And don't forget to drink plenty of water to wash them down the diverticular obstacle course.

DRY MOUTH

Do loud mouths get dry mouths? Unfortunately, dry mouth isn't caused just by yapping too much or too loud, although you can run your throat and vocal chords ragged. Dry mouth, also known as xerostomia, is a condition in which saliva production shuts down.

When working at full capacity, saliva has many duties. This versatile fluid helps us talk, chew, and spit. It acts as a natural cavity fighter by washing away food particles and plaque, and it lubricates food, works to buffer acids, and re-mineralizes those pearly whites. Saliva is vital in maintaining a healthy mouth, so when production decreases or stops, there is more than a dry mouth to pout about. Teeth and gums become more prone to decay and infection, and your taste buds might suffer in their taste-testing abilities.

WHAT CAUSES DRY MOUTH?

Dry mouth is caused by several factors, most commonly by the use of medications. Look on almost any label of nonprescription and prescription drugs, and you'll find that dry mouth is typically listed as a possible side effect. Some of the worst offenders are those drugs designed to dry out your mucous membranes, such as antihistamines and many allergy medications. Other drugs contributing to dryness are those used to treat high blood pressure, depression, and heart disease.

Dehydration is an obvious cause of dry mouth. However, dehydration doesn't always arise from obvious reasons, i.e., not drinking eight glasses of H_2O a day. You can become dehydrated through fever, extensive exercise, vomiting, diarrhea, burns, and blood loss.
Other causes of xerostomia are radiation therapy, menopause, surgical removal of the salivary glands, and cigarette smoking.

The primary symptom of xerostomia is, of course, a dry mouth. But this can be punctuated by myriad other conditions, including excessive thirst, a raw tongue, lip sores, difficulty swallowing, sore throat and hoarseness, bad breath, difficulty speaking, dry nasal passages, and dry lips.

But here's something to smile about: Most cases of dry mouth are easy to solve.

BLAME IT ON YOUR BIRTHDAY

Dry mouth is associated with aging. An estimated 25 to 40 percent of Americans older than 65 suffer from dry mouth.

KITCHEN CURES

ANISEED. Munching on aniseed can help combat the bad breath that accompanies dry mouth. In fact, many Indian restaurants have a bowl of anise and fennel available to remove pungent food odors from your breath. Mix a few teaspoons of these seeds, place in a covered bowl, and keep on the table.

CAYENNE PEPPER. A dry mouth often inhibits taste buds from distinguishing between sour, sweet, salty, and bitter flavors. A mouthwatering method to stimulate saliva production and bolster those buds is to sprinkle red pepper (cayenne) on your food or mix it into your favorite juice (tomato juice seems most compatible). Better yet, prepare an entire meal around red pepper, which acts as nature's wake-up call, stimulating salivary glands, sweat glands, and tear ducts. Go south of the border with some spicy salsas or make that all-American favorite, chili, and start drooling!

CELERY. If you need an excuse to snack, here it is! Munching on such waterlogged snacks as celery sticks helps stimulate the saliva glands and adds moisture to your mouth. Should your sweet tooth strike, suck on sugarless candies. Definitely stay away from sugar-filled treats since they promote decay in an already vulnerable mouth.

FENNEL. Munching on fennel seeds mixed with aniseed can help combat bad breath that accompanies dry mouth. In addition, fennel seed can be combined with other herbs to make a mouthwash.

LIQUIDS. If the salivary glands are down for the count, you'll need all the reinforcements you can muster to help get food down. Try to complement each dish with sauce, gravy, broth, butter, or yogurt. Food will be easier to swallow. Another option is to stick to soft, liquidy foods, such as stews, soups, and noodle dishes.

PARSLEY. A dry mouth is not only uncomfortable, but it often brings out bad breath. This double whammy can ruin just about any social situation. Luckily, battling bad breath is easy. See that parsley on your plate? The restaurant may put it there for decoration, but it can serve a more useful purpose. This herb is a natural breath sweetener, and it provides ample amounts of vitamins A and C, calcium, and iron. So, chew on some.

ROSEMARY. Store-bought mouthwash overflows with germ-killing alcohol, which is also a drying agent. Read labels and don't purchase any that contain alcohol. Better yet, reach into your spice rack and pull out rosemary, mint, and aniseed to make a refreshing herbal mouthwash. The rosemary helps fight germs, while the mint and aniseed freshen breath. Combine 1 teaspoon dried rosemary, 1 teaspoon dried mint, and 1 teaspoon aniseed with 2 $1/2$ cups boiling water. Cover and steep for 15 to 20 minutes. Strain and refrigerate. Use as a gargle.

WATER. Tap or bottled, whatever way you drink water is fine...just drink plenty of it. To keep your system well lubricated, it's recommended you down eight, 8-ounce glasses each day. Cut back on other refreshments such as coffee, sugary sodas, and alcohol, all of which can exacerbate dry mouth. Make sure to accompany every meal with a glass of water.

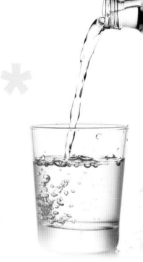

RESTORING ELECTROLYTES

Since dehydration is a major cause of dry mouth, it is vital to restore electrolytes to the body. This kitchen-made elixir works like a commercial sports drink but is much less expensive and doesn't require a trip to the grocery store. Mix 1 teaspoon salt, $1/2$ teaspoon baking soda, and 1 tablespoon sugar into a cup of water. Mix in a dash of lemon, lime, or orange for added flavor. Drink 1 cup a day or more following heavy exercise, vomiting, or a bad case of diarrhea.

NOT JUST FOR COLDS

Echinacea, an herb that's recently been touted as a remedy for colds and flu, also contains a saliva stimulant. Unfortunately, echinacea isn't famous for making a tasty tea, so try disguising the taste. Mix a dropperful of echinacea tincture into your favorite juice (several times per day if necessary). Or, if it's available, chew the root of the fresh plant. Just don't expect to find it delicious.

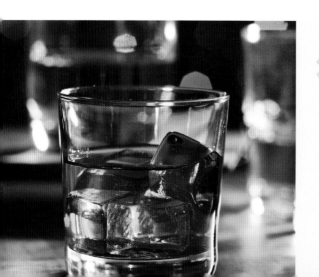

DRINKS TO AVOID

Cut down on coffee and alcohol consumption. Both are diuretics and can leave your mouth feeling as dry as the Sahara.

FATIGUE

Americans are all too familiar with being tired. Polls repeatedly show that many adults don't get eight hours of sleep a night, the amount that's recommended for good health and safety. Many even get less than seven hours a night during the work week.

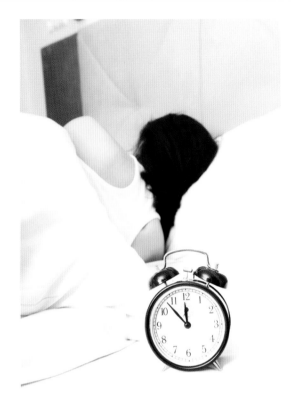

Not getting enough sleep is sure to contribute to fatigue, but what people are doing while they're awake is another problem. Many Americans work more than 50 hours a week. People are spending less time taking care of themselves—sitting down to read a good book, going for a bike ride with the kids, eating a healthy meal. The bottom line: Most people are exhausted. In fact, ten million Americans will visit their doctors this year and ask the same question, "Why am I so tired?"

WHAT TYPE OF TIRED ARE YOU?

There are two types of fatigue: emotional and physical. Emotional fatigue is a tiredness of the mind. It happens when stress piles up, such as having to meet multiple deadlines at work or dealing with the unexpected death of a parent. Physical fatigue happens when you spend the day working in the garden and at the end of the day you can't even lift your little toe. Both types of tiredness can cause you to feel lethargic. And they both require rest and relaxation. How do you know what type of tired you're experiencing? If you wake up tired in the morning but start feeling better as the day goes on, take a look at what's going on in your life emotionally. The key to your fatigue may be in your head. If the morning finds you energized and raring to go, but you start to lose your spark as the afternoon appears, you're probably dealing with a physical problem.

REASONS FOR EMOTIONAL FATIGUE:

- **Doing too much.** You're a room mother, a Girl Scout leader, and now you've decided to take on the school's annual fund drive. And you wonder why you're wiped out?

- **Doing too little.** Sounds strange, but boredom makes you tired. Being motivated to accomplish goals adds a spark to your life. The secret is finding the right balance.

- **Stressful situations.** Major turmoil such as changing jobs or moving to a new city can make you feel exhausted.

- **Mental maladies.** People who are lonely or depressed are prone to tiredness.

REASONS FOR PHYSICAL FATIGUE:

- **Skipping needed nutrients.** Low-calorie diets, fasting, or just missing meals because of meetings or too-busy schedules can wipe you out.

- **Not sleeping enough.** There's no perfect number of hours you should sleep. Different people have different sleep needs. But if you wake up feeling exhausted morning after morning, you might need to add a few more sleeping hours in your day.

- **Getting no exercise.** Exercise is essential to feeling better—physically and mentally.

- **Dodging drinks.** Dehydration is an energy zapper. Drinking and eating go hand-in-hand in giving your body the fuel it needs to feel good.

FATIGUE AS A SYMPTOM OF DISEASE

Fatigue that is brought on by an unexpected loss of sleep, like being a new parent, or a stressful situation, like being a new parent, is usually easily remedied simply by taking good care of yourself. But ongoing fatigue can be the signal that something more serious is going on in your body. **It can often be a symptom of:**

- Anemia
- Arthritis
- A slower-than-usual thyroid (hypothyroidism)
- An underlying sleep disorder
- Cancer
- Chronic fatigue syndrome
- Diabetes
- Heart disease

Talk to your doctor about your symptoms if you're experiencing fatigue. And boost your immune system and health by adding in nutrients.

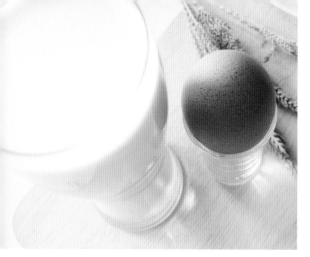

KITCHEN CURES

COFFEE. Caffeine is a known pick-me-up. And the American Dietetic Association says there's no harm in drinking the stimulating stuff, as long as you do so in moderation. Studies confirm that caffeine does perk up the brain and get those mental faculties humming. But be careful—the ADA says a couple of cups a day should do you fine. More than that and you risk anxiety and insomnia.

EGGS. This is a folk remedy that is backed by sound nutrition. One of the most important ways you can battle fatigue is to eat a well-balanced diet, and eggs are loaded with good things such as protein, iron, vitamin A, folic acid, riboflavin, and pantothenic acid. Eat one egg a day, however you like it, and you may be feeling better in no time.

FLUIDS. Drink plenty of water, juice, milk, or other beverages to keep yourself hydrated. Dehydration can contribute to fatigue.

GINSENG. Ginseng is an age-old energy booster. This root has a sweet licorice taste and has been used for thousands of years to treat weakness and exhaustion. Be cautious: Don't take ginseng unless you are really fatigued. It can be too stimulating if you're feeling fine. In America you're probably wise to buy Asian ginseng. Another variety, Siberian ginseng, may not be as potent as the Asian variety. Both Asian and Siberian ginseng varieties of the herb have been labeled "adaptogens." That means they help you adapt to stresses in your environment. You can buy ginseng powder at a reputable herb shop. Take 2 grams of ginseng powder a day for a six-week stint. Then take at least a two-week break before using the energizing herb again.

SKIM MILK. Mixing a little protein with your carbohydrates can keep you energized. Eating only carbohydrates, such as a doughnut or a pancake slathered in syrup, can cause serotonin, a neurotransmitter, to build up in the brain, making you feel drowsy. Eating protein with your carbohydrates can block that sleepy feeling and leave you feeling energized. A good meal to start your day—cereal covered with a good dousing of skim milk.

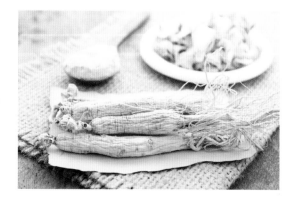

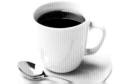

FEVER

Fever is a good thing. It's your body's attempt to kill off invading bacteria and other nasty organisms that can't survive the heat. The hypothalamus, which is the body's thermostat, senses the assault on the body and turns up the heat much the way you turn up the thermostat when you feel cold. It's a simple defense mechanism, and the sweat that comes with a fever is merely a way to cool the body down.

It used to be standard medical practice to knock that fever out as quickly as possible. Not so anymore. The value of fever is recognized, and since a fever will usually subside when the infection that's causing it runs its course, modern thinking is to ride out that fever, especially if it stays under 102°F in adults. However, if a fever is making you uncomfortable or interfering with your ability to eat, drink, or sleep, treat it. Your body needs adequate nutrition, hydration, and rest to fight the underlying cause of the fever.

Fever is a symptom, not an illness, and so there's no specific cure. But there are some fever-relievers in the kitchen that may make you feel better for the duration. Be aware that the most significant side effect of fever is dehydration. Specific ways to deal with it can be found in the Dehydration profile, pages 52–56.

KITCHEN CURES

APPLE WATER. It tastes good, relieves the miseries of fever, and keeps the body hydrated. To make it, peel, skin, core, and slice 3 sweet apples. Put them in a pan with 3 ¾ cups water. Bring to a boil, then simmer until the apples are barely mushy. Remove, strain without pressing apple puree into the liquid, and add 2 tablespoons honey. Drink and enjoy.

BASIL. Mix 1 teaspoon basil with ¼ teaspoon black pepper. Steep in 1 cup hot water to make a tea. Add 1 teaspoon honey. Drink two to three times a day.

BLACKBERRY VINEGAR. This is a great fever elixir, but it takes several days to prepare. Pour cider vinegar over a pound or two of blackberries, then cover the container and store it in a cool, dark place for three days. Strain for a day, since it takes time for all the liquid to drain from the berries, and collect the liquid in another container. Then add 2 cups sugar to each 2 ½ cups juice. Bring to a boil, then simmer for 5 minutes while you skim the scum off the top. Cool and store in an airtight jar in a cool place. Mix 1 teaspoonful with water to quench the thirst caused by a fever.

CILANTRO (coriander leaves). Nice, fresh cilantro can be turned into a simple fever remedy. Wash thoroughly and place a handful of leaves in a blender with $1/3$ cup water. Blend thoroughly, then strain, reserving the liquid. Take 2 teaspoons of the liquid three times a day.

CREAM OF TARTAR. Try this fever tea. Combine $1 \frac{1}{2}$ teaspoons cream of tartar, $1/2$ teaspoon lemon juice, $2 \frac{1}{2}$ cups warm water, and $1/2$ teaspoon honey. Drink 4 to 6 ounces at a time.

GINGER. This can help break a high fever. Grate 2 tablespoons fresh ginger and add to 2 cups boiling water. Steep 30 minutes. Add a little honey to sweeten, and drink a cup of the warm beverage every two to three hours.

FRUIT JUICE. It will replace the fluids lost through sweating. Lemonade is a good choice, too.

LETTUCE. Pour a pint of boiling water over an entire head of lettuce and let it steep, covered, for 15 minutes. Strain, sweeten the liquid to taste, and drink. In addition to keeping you hydrated, this lettuce infusion may help you sleep better.

OREGANO. A tea made from a mixture of some spice rack staples can help reduce fever. Steep 1 teaspoon each of oregano and marjoram in a pint of boiling water for 30 minutes. Strain, and drink warm a couple times a day. Refrigerate unused portion until needed, then gently warm.

PINEAPPLE. Fresh is best. It's one of nature's anti-inflammatory agents that can fight fever. Pineapple is also packed with juice that can prevent dehydration.

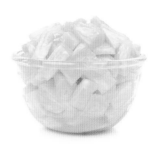

POPSICLE. These can reduce the risk of dehydration. Fruit juice bars are good, too. This can be an especially handy way to keep fluids in small children.

RAISINS. Drink a little of this several times a day to keep yourself hydrated during a fever. Put $3/4$ cup chopped raisins in $7 \frac{1}{2}$ cups water. Bring to a boil, then simmer until the water has been reduced by one-third.

SAGE. Mix 2 teaspoons dried sage with 1 teaspoon dried peppermint. Pour 1 cup boiling water over these and steep 15 minutes. Strain and sweeten with honey. Drink 2 to 3 cups per day, rewarmed. Add a little honey to sweeten the taste.

WATER. Drink lots of it to prevent dehydration. Sponging the body with lukewarm water can relieve fever symptoms, but it's recommended that you use fever-reducing medication first to reduce the possibility of chills and shivering. Do not use cold water or ice on the body.

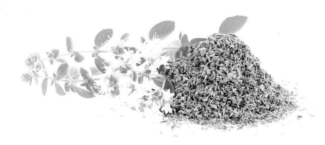

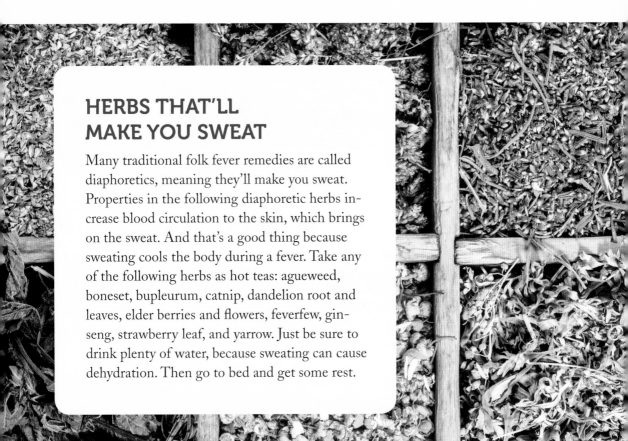

HERBS THAT'LL MAKE YOU SWEAT

Many traditional folk fever remedies are called diaphoretics, meaning they'll make you sweat. Properties in the following diaphoretic herbs increase blood circulation to the skin, which brings on the sweat. And that's a good thing because sweating cools the body during a fever. Take any of the following herbs as hot teas: agueweed, boneset, bupleurum, catnip, dandelion root and leaves, elder berries and flowers, feverfew, ginseng, strawberry leaf, and yarrow. Just be sure to drink plenty of water, because sweating can cause dehydration. Then go to bed and get some rest.

MORE DO'S & DON'TS

- Skip the alcohol and caffeine. They're diuretics, and you don't need to lose more fluid.

- If you don't feel like eating, don't, even though your mother told you to feed that fever and starve that cold. Just make sure you get sufficient fluids. Do reintroduce yourself to foods gradually, though, if you haven't been eating very much.

FIBROCYSTIC BREAST DISEASE

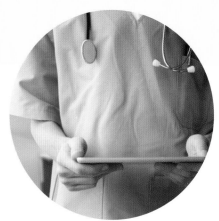

Although the term fibrocystic breast disease may sound ominous, it actually describes a benign condition of the breasts that more than 60 percent of all women experience. If your breasts feel lumpy and you have intermittent breast discomfort, such as tenderness, swelling, and pain, you may have fibrocystic breast disease.

How can you tell? Symptoms include a dense, irregular, and bumpy consistency of the breast tissue. During a self-exam, you may feel a thick area of irregularly shaped tissue with a lumpy or ridgelike surface, or you may encounter a beadlike texture to your breast tissue. Fibrocystic breasts typically become swollen, tender, heavy, and lumpier a week or two before the menstrual period. There also may be changes in nipple sensation, and the nipples may itch. These symptoms can range from mild to severe, and they usually improve after menstruation. Some women, however, have persistent rather than intermittent symptoms. The condition tends to subside with menopause.

WHAT'S BEHIND THE PAIN...AND WHAT'S NOT

No one understands the causes of this condition, but some researchers believe that breast lumps are inherited. What we do know is that the condition is related to how the breast responds to hormonal changes during the monthly cycle. Hormonal stimulation causes milk glands and ducts to swell and the breast to retain water. The condition is more common in women aged 30 to 50, most likely because of years of repeated hormonal stimulation, which can harden lumps.

What's usually not behind the pain is breast cancer. Only five percent of fibrocystic conditions have the type of changes that would be considered a risk factor for developing breast cancer, according to the American Cancer Society. Unlike the lumps associated with fibrocystic breast disease, which are tender and move freely, cancerous lumps most often are not tender and don't move freely.

If you think you have fibrocystic breast disease, be sure to check it out with your physician, who should always examine any lump(s) in the breast. You'll be pleased to discover that breast tenderness and other symptoms can often be managed through diet.

KITCHEN CURES

FISH. The best fish for female health include those high in the omega-3 fatty acids such as salmon, trout, and mackerel. These fish are also high in iodine, a deficiency of which may be a factor in the development of breast lumps. Eating moderate amounts of fish may help prevent lumps.

KELP. Kelp and other sea vegetables, such as nori and dulse, are good sources of iodine. Studies suggest that an iodine deficiency can predispose women to having breast lumps. While you can find these vegetables in some food markets, kelp and dulce are also available in powdered form and can be used in cooking as a salt substitute.

VEGETABLES. Diuretics help flush excess fluids from the body and reduce breast swelling. Unfortunately, many store-bought diuretics can also deplete your potassium reserves, unbalance your electrolyte count, and interfere with glucose production. Turn to natural diuretics instead. Parsley, cucumbers, and cabbage are healthy for you and will keep you naturally flushed.

WHOLE-GRAIN FOODS. Increasing your intake of fiber can help control the hormonal fluctuations behind fibrocystic breast disease. Eat whole-wheat bread, brown rice, beans, and fruits.

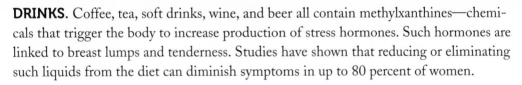

* FOODS TO AVOID *

DRINKS. Coffee, tea, soft drinks, wine, and beer all contain methylxanthines—chemicals that trigger the body to increase production of stress hormones. Such hormones are linked to breast lumps and tenderness. Studies have shown that reducing or eliminating such liquids from the diet can diminish symptoms in up to 80 percent of women.

MEATS. Cut back on meat consumption. Before heading to the butcher's block, consider that cows, chicken, and other livestock are often pumped full of hormones. Your body doesn't need the additional influx, especially during the hormone high time of your period. If meat needs to be on the menu, purchase hormone-free meats and poultry at a health food store.

SALT. Two weeks before your period, hide the saltshaker. During the menstrual cycle, women tend to retain water, which in turn causes their breasts to feel heavy and become sensitive. Salt only increases this uncomfortable bloating. Be aware of the hidden salts in processed foods, too, and save that pizza order until after your period.

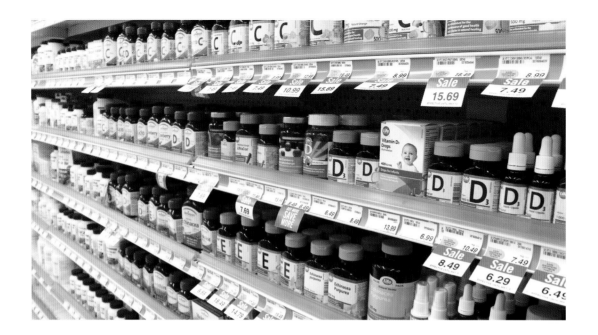

FROM THE SUPPLEMENT SHELF

ESSENTIAL FATTY ACIDS. Several studies have looked at the beneficial effects of evening primrose oil on fibrocystic breast disease. Evening primrose oil is an excellent source of the essential fatty acid linolenic acid and its chemical derivative, gamma linolenic acid (GLA). Typical dosages used in the studies were 1,500 mg twice a day. (This would amount to taking 6 of the 500 mg capsules commonly available at health food stores.) Borage oil and black currant oil are more concentrated sources of GLA, so you need to take fewer capsules. For example, 3 or 4 capsules per day of borage oil may be sufficient. However, always discuss dosages with your physician before taking any of these oils.

VITAMIN A/BETA-CAROTENE. Some studies have shown that vitamin A can reduce breast pain in women with moderate to severe symptoms. There is a risk to taking high doses of vitamin A, however, because it can be toxic. It's safer to eat a diet high in beta carotene, the precursor to vitamin A, with yellow, orange, red, and dark green vegetables and fruits.

VITAMIN E. In several controlled studies, vitamin E was found to be quite helpful in reducing the pain and tenderness, as well as the size, of breast lumps. Vitamin E can be found in vegetable oils, nuts, green leafy vegetables, and some fortified cereals. Or you can take a daily supplement.

FLATULENCE

Who is the most glamorous person you know? Well, guess what. That person's not exempt from this particular problem. No one is. And it happens at the most awkward times, doesn't it? You feel that rumble way down deep in your belly, and it's traveling even lower. In the middle of very polite—and very quiet—company it gurgles inside, and you glance at the person next to you so no one will know that the undertone of the impending blast belongs to you.

Well, gas happens. Called flatus, or flatulence when it finally does escape, it's normal. Its beginnings are in the foods we eat. We eat, therefore we pass gas. Why? Our stomach acids are breaking down last night's pasta primavera into elements that will either be absorbed into the body or eliminated. And that breakdown causes…You guessed it: Gas!

Bodily gas originates in the stomach and travels down to the intestines (unless it comes back up as a belch). Its construction is pretty simple: carbon dioxide, hydrogen, nitrogen, and methane. Well, those gases make up about 99 percent of the gas we pass. The other 1 percent is divided among up to 250 different gases, all of which occur naturally when carbohydrates are broken down. If you swallow air, you add oxygen to the mix.

Here are some other interesting flatus facts:

- Normal flatus production is 6 to 64 ounces each day.
- There are 400 different kinds of bacteria living in your colon, waiting to mix and mingle with your food and give you gas.
- We pass gas, on average, 14 to 23 times each day.

Gas normally has no odor, unless you're squeezed into the elevator with the people who ate beans for dinner last night. Then the eye-watering "squeakers" they're responsible for are enough to make you haul out the old gas mask. The reason: Some foods simply hang around in the intestines too long and begin to ferment. Fermentation causes the offensive odor. And the more food that's fermenting, the more volume of gas building up for its grand exit.

WHO'S PRONE

There are a few factors that make you more prone to passing gas. **See if you're on the list:**

- Anyone who dines regularly on the flatulogenic food list. See page 96.

- Those with certain stomach intestinal ailments, such as lactose intolerance or irritable bowel syndrome.

- Air-swallowers

- Those with gassy relatives. The tendency can be inherited.

- Anyone with food allergies that manifest in flatus after certain foods are eaten

- Gas is a side effect or symptom, not an illness in itself. And it's a symptom that can be treated several different ways with things you find in the kitchen.

NOTING *
IT DOWN *

Keep a food diary and list the foods that are causing your gas. Include such information as the type of food, when you ate it, and how much you ate. Do you get gassy after gulping down cucumbers or cola? Or maybe it happens after eating ice cream? (See Lactose Intolerance, page 144.) The truth about most gas is that, in some way, you're causing it. If you want to find out how, a food diary is one of the easiest ways to recreate the events leading up to the noxious crime.

KITCHEN CURES

CARAWAY CRACKERS. Caraway seeds and their oils are carminatives (they get rid of gas), but who wants to eat just the seeds? Caraway seed crackers and breads with caraway seeds are a tasty way to make your system gas-unfriendly.

CARDAMOM SEEDS. These speed digestion. Add them to sautéed vegetables or to rice or lentils before cooking. You can also chew whole pods or steep pods in boiling water for several minutes to make a tea.

CLOVES. They pep up digestion and eliminate gas. Add 2 to 3 whole cloves to rice before cooking. Sprinkle on apples and pears when baking. Or steep 2 to 3 whole cloves in a cup of boiling water for ten minutes, sweeten to taste, and drink.

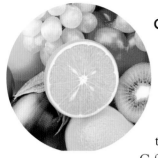

CITRUS FRUITS. Vitamin C in tablet form may cause gas, especially amounts in excess of 500 milligrams. So, reduce the dosage and replace the C with these high-in-C fruits. Also try the following vegetables, which are high in vitamin C: potatoes, sweet peppers.

CORIANDER. This helps in the downward movement of foods being digested and can ease cramps, hiccups, bloating, and flatulence. Crush the seeds into powder and add to foods such as vegetable stir-fry. Its flavor really enhances curry and Middle Eastern dishes, too.

FENNEL SEEDS. It's an acquired taste, but it may be one well worth acquiring if you're plagued by gas. Fennel's digestive powers are so good that in India fennel is customarily eaten after a meal to help digestion and freshen the breath. For gas, drink it as a tea by steeping ½ teaspoon seeds in 1 cup boiling water for ten minutes. Or, sprinkle them over those gassy vegetables during cooking or add to stir-fries. If you've acquired the taste, fennel also works well cooked into figs, apples, pears, and plums.

GINGER. Combine 1 teaspoon fresh grated ginger with 1 teaspoon lime juice. Take after eating.

LEMON. Stir 1 teaspoon lemon juice and ½ teaspoon baking soda into 1 cup cool water. Skip the ice water; it can start digestive spasms that cause gas. Drink after meals.

PUMPKIN. It soothes the tummy, and best of all, it cuts down on flatulence. Try some baked, steamed, or broiled. Or, make yourself a simple pumpkin soup.

ROSEMARY. If you're eating a gassy food, sprinkle on a little rosemary to cut down the effect. You can do the same with sage and thyme, too.

TEA HERBS. Steep and drink a tea made from any of these: aniseed, basil leaves, chamomile, cloves, cinnamon, ginger, peppermint, sage. Steep about ½ teaspoon in 1 cup boiling water, then add honey or lemon to taste. Drink one to three times each day.

TURMERIC. This may stop a gas problem altogether. Turmeric is one of the many flavorful and curative spices found in curry powder. You can add turmeric itself to rice or season a bland dish with curry powder, which contains turmeric. However you use it, it helps alleviate gas.

YOGURT WITH ACIDOPHILUS. It alleviates digestive woes, including gas. But the yogurt must have live acidophilus, a bacteria that helps with digestion.

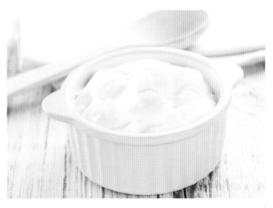

MORE DO'S & DON'TS

- Try cutting back some on fiber, especially from legumes. Fiber is good for you, but increasing fiber intake too quickly can cause gas.

- Reduce the amount of fermented foods you eat, such as cheese, soy sauce, and alcohol.

- Cut back on carbonated beverages.

- Don't stuff yourself when you eat. The more food in the gut, the more gas buildup. And eat more slowly—you'll swallow less air.

- Don't sip drinks through a straw. You'll suck in air, which causes gas.

FLATULOGENIC FOODS

If you're plagued by gas, here are some foods that are definitely on the top of the flatus-maker list:

Beer	Carbonated drinks	Milk
Bran	Cauliflower	Onions
Broccoli	Corn	Rutabaga
Brussels sprouts	Legumes	
Cabbage	(beans, lentils, dried peas)	

These are also gas-making culprits:

Apples	Cucumbers	Raisins
Apricots	Eggplant	Soybeans
Bananas	Lettuce	Spinach
Carrots	Melon	Strawberries
Celery	Potatoes	Wheat products
Citrus fruits	Prunes	
Coffee	Radishes	

THINKING ABOUT GIVING THOSE BEANS THE BOOT?

Don't do it! Beans are loaded with cholesterol-lowering fiber and bone-saving calcium, and they have a hand in protecting against colon cancer and heart disease. So instead of bagging the beans, find out which ones cause you the most trouble and boot those out of your diet. Pintos, black beans, and Great Northerns are generally the biggest gas-makers. What's gassy for some, though, may not be gassy for others. It's all a matter of how your body digests them.

If you love them but they don't love you back, there's a simple solution to eliminate most of the gas-causing effects.

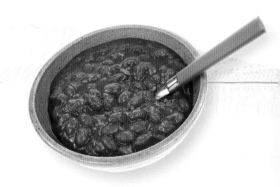

1. Soak beans in water overnight.
2. Replace the water with fresh water and cook the beans for 30 minutes. Drain the water again.
3. Add fresh water and cook for another 30 minutes. Drain the water one more time.
4. Add fresh water and cook until done.

And, if you like the flavor of onion in those beans, skip the fresh onions. They share their gassy juices with everything that's in the bean pot. Instead, opt for dehydrated onions that will absorb the liquid already there instead of adding to it.

You can also keep Beano sitting right next to that bag of dry beans to remind you it's a gas-busting enzyme that breaks down hard-to-digest disaccharides, thereby avoiding the formation of gas. Use this product as you eat the gassy foods, not afterward. It's available at groceries and pharmacies.

PRESSURE
COOKING POWER

Beans that are undercooked are more likely to cause gas than beans that are well-cooked. To ensure that your beans are cooked thoroughly, pull out the pressure cooker and follow the manufacturer's advice for cooking beans. Or, cook them up to pressure for 30 minutes at 15 pounds per square inch on the gauge.

97

FLU (INFLUENZA)

Boo hoo if you've got the flu. Unlike the common cold, which causes a stuffy nose, sore throat, and sneezing, the flu is a viral infection that strikes the entire body with a vengeance. The misery starts suddenly with chills and fever and spirals into more unpleasant symptoms that will take you out of commission: a sore throat, dry cough, stuffy or runny nose, headache, nausea, vomiting, severe muscle aches and pains, weakness, backache, and loss of appetite. Some people even experience pain and stiffness in the joints.

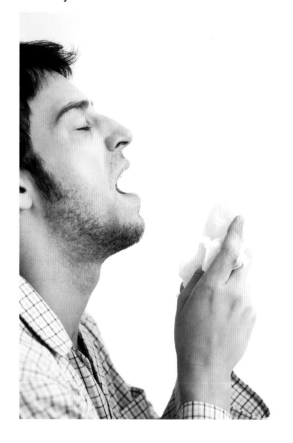

The worst of your symptoms will last about three to five days, but others, such as cough and fatigue, can linger for weeks. And a bout with the flu can deliver a double whammy if you develop a secondary infection, such as an ear or sinus infection or bronchitis. Even pneumonia can be a complication—and a potentially serious one—of influenza.

Flu viruses strike like clockwork in the United States. Every year they begin to show up in October and exit in April. Peak flu season is December and January.

Flu is a highly contagious illness, spread by droplets from the respiratory tract of an infected person. These can be airborne, such as those released after a person coughs or sneezes, or they can be transferred via an infected person's hands.

Taking a yearly flu shot can help you ward off infection, and these are particularly recommended for senior citizens, people with compromised immune systems, or people with asthma. They won't give you 100 percent protection, but they will significantly increase your chances of avoiding it.

If you do get the flu, there are kitchen remedies to help ease your suffering.

KITCHEN CURES

BROTH. Canned broth, whether it's beef, chicken, or vegetable, will keep you hydrated and help liquefy any mucous secretions. Broth is easy to keep down, even when you have no appetite, and will provide at least some nutrients.

HONEY. A hacking cough can keep you and every other household member up all night. Keep the peace with honey. Honey has long been used in traditional medicine for coughs. It's a simple enough recipe: Mix 1 tablespoon honey into 1 cup hot water, stir well, and enjoy. Honey acts as a natural expectorant, promoting the flow of mucus. Squeeze some lemon in if you want a little tartness.

JUICE. Any flavor or kind will do. Just drink lots of juice both to keep yourself hydrated and to give yourself some extra vitamins.

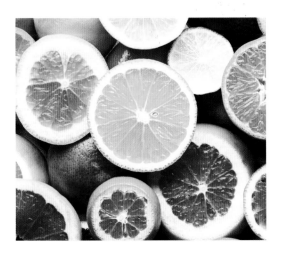

LEMON. The lovely lemon may cause a puckered face if eaten raw, but in a hot beverage lemons will have you smiling. Hot lemonade has been used as a flu remedy since Roman times and is still highly regarded in the folk traditions of New England. Lemons, being highly acidic, help make mucous membranes distasteful to bacteria and viruses. Lemon oil, which gives the juice its fragrance, is like a wonder drug containing antibacterial, antiviral, antifungal, and anti-inflammatory constituents. The oil also acts as an expectorant. To make this flu-fighting fruit drink, place 1 chopped lemon—skin, pulp, and all—into 1 cup boiling water. While the lemon steeps for 5 minutes, inhale the steam. Strain, add honey (to taste), and enjoy. Drink hot lemonade three to four times a day throughout your illness.

PEPPER. Pepper is an irritant (try sniffling some), yet this annoying characteristic is a plus for those suffering from coughs with thick mucus. The irritating property of pepper stimulates circulation and the flow of mucus. Place 1 teaspoon black pepper into a cup and sweeten things up with the addition of 1 tablespoon honey. Fill with boiling water, let steep for 10 to 15 minutes, stir, and sip.

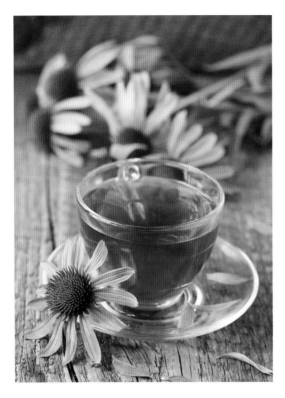

TEA. A cup of hot tea is just another way to take your fluids, which are so essential when you have the flu. Just be sure to choose decaffeinated varieties. Caffeine is a mild diuretic, which is counterproductive when you have the flu, and you certainly don't want to be awakened with the need to use the bathroom when you need your rest!

THYME. It's time to try thyme when the mucous membranes are stuffed, the head aches, and the body is hot with fever. Wonderfully fragrant, thyme delights the senses (if you can smell when sick) and works as a powerful expectorant and antiseptic, thanks to its constituent oil, thymol. By cupping your hands around a mug of thyme tea and breathing in the steam, the thymol sets to work through your upper respiratory tract, loosening mucus and inhibiting bacteria from settling down to stay. Make thyme tea in a snap by adding 1 teaspoon dried thyme leaves to 1 cup boiling water. Let steep for five minutes while inhaling the steam. Strain the tea, sweeten with honey (to taste), and slowly sip.

FIGHT FLU
WITH FLUIDS

- Drink lots of fluids. Water's good, as are teas, juice, and soups. Off-limits are coffee and soda pop, as they may contain caffeine and have no nutritional benefits whatsoever.

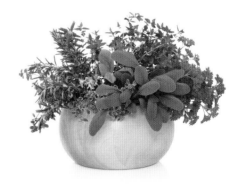

HERBAL REMEDIES

You may not ordinarily keep these herbs in your kitchen, but it's a good idea to stock up on them before flu seasons starts. Then you can put together some soothing remedies for influenza symptoms.

Lemon Balm. For adults who can't catch their *zzz*'s while coping with the flu, lemon balm acts as a mild sedative. It also contains antiviral compounds to help disinfect mucous membranes. To make this relaxing potion, place 1 teaspoon dried lemon balm in 1 cup boiling water. Cover and let steep for ten minutes. Strain, sweeten with honey (to taste), and drink up to 4 cups a day. (Note: Lemon balm is also known as balm mint, bee balm, blue balm, garden balm, Melissa, and sweet balm.)

Peppermint. Running a fever of 102°F to 104°F is common with the flu. A way to cool your hot head, via sweating, is with a cup of peppermint tea. As an added bonus, peppermint contains menthol, which works as a decongestant to help unstuff sinuses. And peppermint has antispasmodic properties to help that hack. To make this fever fighter, place ½ ounce peppermint leaves in a 1-quart jar of boiling water. Cover and let steep 20 minutes. Strain the liquid, add a cube of sugar if you'd like, and enjoy 2 to 3 cups a day.

Thyme and Peppermint. Variety is the spice of life! Combine thyme and peppermint to make an herbal steam broth that will deliver healing aromas to your aching nose and throat. Combine 1 ½ quarts boiling water and 2 tablespoons each of dried thyme and peppermint in a large pot. Cover and steep for five minutes. Place the pot on a table and remove the lid. Lean in and cover both your head and the pot of steaming herbs with a large towel. Slowly breathe the herbal broth for 15 minutes. **(Warning: Don't stick your nose too close to the broth or you'll risk a burn.)**

FOOD POISONING

The company's annual 4th of July barbecue started out a huge success. The ribs were superb. The potato salad was excellent. Even Helen's famous coleslaw got rave reviews. But about the time the sun went down, people started sprinting in all directions, and they weren't running in the three-legged race. Most of them were headed for the nearest bathroom. Food poisoning claims another round of victims.

The Centers for Disease Control and Prevention estimates that there will be about 76 million cases of food poisoning this year. It's an estimate because most cases of food poisoning go unreported, chalked up to the stomach flu or another bug. Even though the United States has strict guidelines when it comes to processing and handling food, there is always a risk of some food becoming contaminated. Ironically, though many cases of food poisoning do happen in restaurants, the most common place for foodborne illnesses to strike is your kitchen.

HOW SPOILED FOOD MAKES YOU FEEL

The symptoms you have after eating a pork chop laden with bad bacteria can range from mild (a few stomach cramps) to severe (you spend a couple of days camped out on the bathroom floor). Many people describe food poisoning as akin to being hit by a very large truck. The most common symptoms are diarrhea, stomach pain, cramping, nausea, and vomiting. Because most of the symptoms of food poisoning are similar to those of other illnesses, such as a stomach virus, people aren't always sure food is the problem. If you think you've got food poisoning but aren't sure, take note: Most people get sick about 4 to 48 hours after eating the suspect food. And if you got sick, chances are everyone else who ate a contaminated chop will be sick, too.

FOILING FOOD POISONING

You've had some potato salad that's been sitting in the sun too long. Your stomach starts to cramp, and you make your first trip to the bathroom. Now what? There's not really anything you can do to stop the symptoms of food poisoning once they start, and you shouldn't try. As awful as it is, the diarrhea and vomiting that happen when you contract a foodborne illness help your body get rid of the poison. Taking over-the-counter medications that halt the process can make you sicker. The best thing you can do is take care of yourself while you're sick. These kitchen remedies can at least make dealing with the symptoms more bearable and get you feeling better faster. There are also some things in your kitchen that will help prevent food poisoning from visiting your house.

KITCHEN CURES

BANANA. As you spend more time embracing the porcelain throne, your body is losing essential elements like potassium. Losing these vital nutrients can make that I've-been-hit-by-a-truck feeling worse. Once you've come to a lull in the bathroom visitations, usually after the first 24 hours, try eating a banana. It's easy on your stomach and can make you feel a bit better.

CHICKEN SOUP. Once you start feeling a bit better, start your stomach out with bland foods. Chicken soup is tasty and easy to digest.

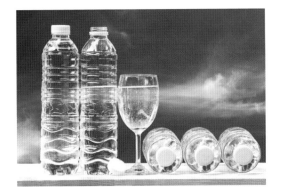

SPORTS DRINKS. Losing all that fluid means you're losing electrolytes (salts that keep your body functioning properly) and water. Replacing that fluid with a sports drink will help replace needed electrolytes, and the sugar in the drink will help your body better absorb the fluid it needs. If the sugar is too much for your tummy, tone the drink down by diluting it with water.

SUGAR. Sugar helps your body hold onto fluid, and adding a spoonful of sugar to a glass of water or a cup of decaffeinated tea may be more palatable if you find sports drinks too sugary.

WATER. You may not feel like having anything pass your lips, but you've got to stay hydrated, especially when you are losing fluids from both ends. Start off with a few sips of this easy-to-swallow liquid and work your way up to more substantial stuff.

MORE DO'S AND DON'TS

- Don't start back on foods that are hard to digest. Give your stomach and your intestines time to recuperate. Stay away from spicy, smoked, fried, or salty foods. Stay away from raw vegetables or rich pastries or candies, and don't drink alcohol.

- Once you're sick, get someone else to go to the kitchen for you. You could be spreading more harmful bacteria and inviting others to share in your suffering.

BACTERIA'S BAD BOYS

There are somewhere around 100 bacteria that can cause food poisoning. **But these are on "Most Wanted" list:**

Campylobacter jejuni. A common cause of foodborne illness, this bacteria is found in raw and undercooked poultry and meat, unpasteurized milk, and untreated water. Cook food properly and clean hands and utensils to kill it.

Clostridium perfringens. Known as the "buffet germ," this bacteria grows fastest in casseroles, stews, and gravies that are held at low or room temperature. Make sure hot foods are kept hot and cold foods cold.

Escherichia coli (E. Coli) 0157:H7. This specific strain of E. coli can cause severe problems. Found mostly in raw or undercooked ground beef or unpasteurized milk, kill this bacteria by cooking food properly.

Salmonella. Found mostly in raw or undercooked meat, poultry, eggs, and fish, and in unpasteurized milk, salmonella is easy to get rid of. Cook foods thoroughly and drink only pasteurized milk.

Staphylococcus aureus. Staph bacteria is found on people (skin, nose, throat) but is spread through contaminated foods. It can't be killed by cooking; avoid this one by keeping hands and kitchen utensils clean.

Vibrio vulnificus. This bacteria is found in raw oysters and raw or undercooked mussels, clams, and whole scallops.

KEEPING BACTERIA AT BAY

Food that's very hot or very cold won't allow bacteria to grow. **Here are the important numbers to know:**

160°F: The food temperature at which you can begin saying "sayonara" to bacteria.

140°F: Foods cooked and held at this temperature won't be free of bacteria, but bacteria will not be able to spread.

125°F: At this temperature, bacteria can survive and a few will grow.

60°F: If risky food is left at this temperature for too long, bacteria will begin to take over.

40°F: The magic temperature at which potentially dangerous bacteria begin to grow.

32°F: Though most bacteria are halted at this temp, some bacteria will grow.

0°F: Bacteria don't die at this frigid temperature, but you can keep them from spreading.

FOOT DISCOMFORT AND ODOR

Overworked and taken for granted; that's the lot of the lowly foot. But feet are a marvelous work of nature and an absolute architectural wonder. Each one of your feet is made up of 26 bones, 33 joints, 107 ligaments, and 31 tendons. Together, they comprise one-quarter of all the bones in your body.

Every day, on average, we take about 10,000 steps. That adds up to four hikes around the planet during a lifetime. And each time a step is taken, the impact of hitting the ground is about four times your body weight. No wonder, then, that 70 percent of us experience foot and ankle problems at some time.

Foot odor, known in the medical profession as bromhidrosis, can be traced to bacteria that find your moist and warm feet, socks, and shoes the perfect place to breed and multiply. Thousands of sweat glands on the soles of the feet produce perspiration composed of water, sodium chloride, fat, minerals, and various acids that are the end products of your body's metabolism. In the presence of certain bacteria (namely those found in dark, damp shoes), these sweaty secretions break down, generating the stench that turns people green.

To fight food discomfort and odor, turn to these kitchen cures.

ASPARAGUS. For swollen feet, look in the veggie drawer for that nice, fresh asparagus you bought. Steam and eat. Asparagus acts as a natural diuretic, which flushes the excess fluid out of your system.

CINNAMON. Cure those cold feet with some nice hot cinnamon tea. Stir a gram of powdered cinnamon into a glass of hot water and steep for 15 minutes. Drink three times a day.

CUMIN. For swollen feet, mix 1/4 teaspoon each of cumin, coriander, and fennel into a cup of hot water and drink two to three times a day.

FOODS. For bloated, uncomfortable feet, here are some foods that can help balance your fluid levels: bananas, which are high in potassium that helps relieve fluid retention, and coffee or tea, both of which are diuretics. You can also turn to poultry and fresh fish, both of which are low in sodium, and yogurt, which can reduce histamine-producing bacteria. Histamine causes fluid retention.

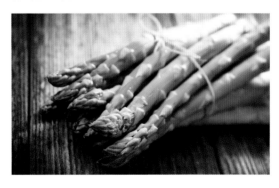

FOODS THAT CAUSE FLUID RETENTION

Sometimes a simple dietary change is all it takes to get rid of those aching swollen feet. **Avoid these foods, which can make your feet puff right up:**

- Bacon and other cured meats. Curing is done with salt, which causes fluid retention.

- Lunch meats. These, too, have lots of salt.

- Canned foods. Salt is added to most canned foods, including vegetables.

FOODS TO WATCH OUT FOR

Watch what foods you eat in abundance. Strong, pungent foods such as garlic, onions, scallions, peppers, and curry spices can cause foot odor. The odoriferous products in each pass through the bloodstream and concentrate in the perspiration.

GALLBLADDER PROBLEMS

Unless you've had problems with your gallbladder, you probably don't know much about it. Be thankful. If you do know the specifics of your gallbladder, you're probably one of the 10 to 15 percent of Americans who have gallstones. While half of those with gallstones experience no symptoms, the other half can have chronic problems, including discomfort and pain in the upper abdomen, indigestion, nausea, and intolerance of fatty foods. A gallbladder attack, which occurs when a gallstone gets stuck in the bile duct, can double you over in pain for hours and leave you wishing something, anything, could make you feel better.

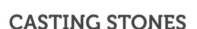

CASTING STONES

The gallbladder is a little pear-shaped pouch tucked behind the lobes of the liver. Its main job is to store up the cholesterol-rich bile that's secreted by the liver. Bile helps your body digest fatty foods. So when that piece of prime rib reaches the intestines, they send a message up to the gallbladder to send some bile their way. Once the bile saturates your steak, it becomes more digestible and easily makes its way through the rest of the digestive process.

At least that's the way things should work. But the reality is that many people, especially older people and women, will have some gallbladder trouble. Ninety percent of the time that trouble is in the form of gallstones. Gallstones form when the bile contains excessive amounts of cholesterol. When there isn't enough bile to saturate the cholesterol, the cholesterol begins to crystallize, and you get a gallstone. These tough bits can be as tiny as a grain of sand or as large as a golf ball. You may not even know you have gallstones unless you happen to have an ultrasound or X ray of your tummy. But the 20 percent of the time that gallstones do cause problems, it's excruciatingly painful.

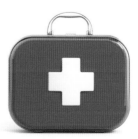

Gallstones become a problem when they get pushed out of the gallbladder and into the tube that connects the liver and the small intestine. The tube gets blocked, and you get 20 minutes to 4 hours of indescribable agony. Pain usually radiates from your upper right abdominal area to your lower right chest, and it can even leave your shoulder and back in agony. Gallstones typically fall back into the gallbladder or make their way through the duct, leaving you feeling better. After you have an attack, you'll probably be sore and wonder what in the world just happened.

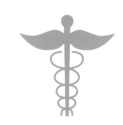

Sometimes, though, the gallstones can get stuck in the bile duct. Symptoms of a stuck gallstone include chills, vomiting, and possibly jaundice in addition to the pain described above.

WHO'S AT RISK?

Pregnancy, obesity, diabetes, liver disease, a sedentary lifestyle, a high fat diet, and certain forms of anemia can all increase the risk of gallstones. People who are overweight and lose and gain weight repeatedly are more susceptible to gallstones, as are women who have had two or more children. Lack of exercise is a significant contributor to the development of gallstones. In fact, according to the Nurses' Health Study, inactivity can actually account for more than half of the risk of developing gallstones. Women are twice as likely as men to develop gallstones, although the reasons are unclear. And people older than 60 years of age have a greater risk of gallstones.

Other risk factors include a family history of gallstones and taking hormones, such as birth control pills or estrogen.

Take heart. There are some specific things you can find in your kitchen to help you avoid a gallstone attack and even prevent gallstones from forming in the first place. What you eat has a great effect on whether or not you develop gallstones. And research is finding that certain foods can help you avert a painful attack or, better yet, avoid gallstones altogether.

KITCHEN CURES

COFFEE. New studies are finding that drinking a couple of cups of java a day can prevent gallstones. One study discovered that men who drank 2 to 3 cups of regular coffee a day cut their risk of developing gallstones by 40 percent. Four cups a day reduced the risk by 45 percent. Researchers are not sure what it is about coffee that helps reduce the risk of forming gallstones, but the effect was the same whether it was cheap, store-bought instant coffee or high-priced espresso. It might be the caffeine; however, teas and soft drinks containing caffeine did not produce the same effect—and neither did decaffeinated coffee.

HIGH-FIBER CEREAL. People who eat a sugary, high-fat diet probably will have more problems with their gallstones. But adding in some fiber-rich foods and avoiding the sugary snacks and fatty foods can help you keep your gallbladder healthy. Grabbing some cereal in the morning will also get something in your tummy. Studies have shown that going for long periods without eating, such as skipping breakfast, can make you more prone to getting a gallstone.

LENTILS. An interesting study found that women who ate loads of lentils, nuts, beans, peas, lima beans, and oranges were more resistant to gallbladder attacks than women who didn't eat much of the stuff.

RED BELL PEPPER. Getting loads of vitamin C in your diet can help you avoid gallstones, and one red bell pepper has 95 mg of the helpful vitamin—more than the 60 mg a day the government recommends for men and women over age 15. A recent study found that people who had more vitamin C in their blood were less likely to get the painful stones.

SALMON. Research is finding that omega-3 fatty acids, found in fatty fish such as salmon, may help prevent gallstones.

VEGETABLES. Eating your veggies is a good way to ward off gallstones. One study found that vegetarian women were only half as likely to have gallstones as their carnivore counterparts. Researchers aren't sure exactly how vegetables counteract gallstones, but they believe vegetables help reduce the amount of cholesterol in bile.

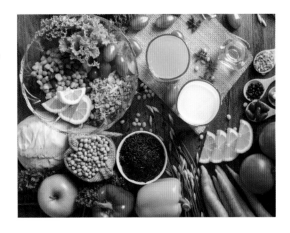

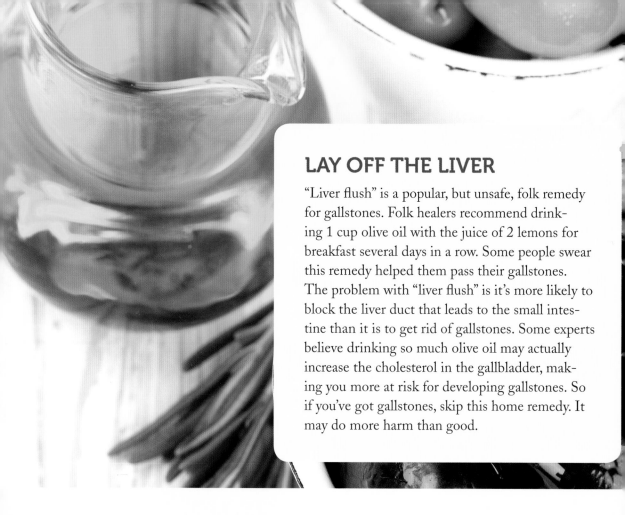

LAY OFF THE LIVER

"Liver flush" is a popular, but unsafe, folk remedy for gallstones. Folk healers recommend drinking 1 cup olive oil with the juice of 2 lemons for breakfast several days in a row. Some people swear this remedy helped them pass their gallstones. The problem with "liver flush" is it's more likely to block the liver duct that leads to the small intestine than it is to get rid of gallstones. Some experts believe drinking so much olive oil may actually increase the cholesterol in the gallbladder, making you more at risk for developing gallstones. So if you've got gallstones, skip this home remedy. It may do more harm than good.

MORE DO'S AND DON'TS

- Lose some weight. Being overweight, even as little as 10 pounds, can double your risk of getting gallstones.

- Diet sensibly. If you are overweight, plan on shedding pounds slowly. Losing weight too fast can increase your chances of developing gallstones.

- Reduce your saturated fat intake. Too much fat in the diet increases your risk of gallstones. But don't cut back too drastically. You need some fat to give the gallbladder the message to empty bile. If you're trying to lose weight, don't go below 20 percent calories from fat.

- Eat a low fat, low-cholesterol, high-fiber diet. Multiple studies show this is your best bet for a healthy body and a healthy gallbladder.

GOUT

The word gout may make you think of kings and medieval history. But gout isn't a disease of the past. It's very much with us today. That's because gout is an inflammatory joint disease and a form of arthritis, not some mysterious illness of the rich and powerful.

Gout, which occurs in about five percent of people with arthritis, results from the buildup of uric acid in the blood. Uric acid is the result of the breakdown of waste substances, called purines, in the body. Usually it is dissolved in the blood, processed by the kidneys, and passed out of the body in the urine. But in some people there is an excess amount of uric acid, too much for the kidneys to eliminate quickly. When there is too much uric acid in the blood, it crystallizes and collects in the joint spaces, causing gout. Occasionally, these deposits become so large that they push against the skin in lumpy patches, called tophi, that can actually be seen.

A gout attack usually lasts five to ten days, and the most common area under siege is the big toe. In fact, 75 percent of people with gout will be affected in the big toe at some time. Gout in the big toe can become so painful that even a bedsheet draped over it will cause intolerable pain. Besides the big toe, gout may also develop in the ankles, heels, knees, wrists, fingers, and elbows.

WHO GETS GOUT?

Though anyone can get gout, it's primarily a man's disease. Women have the good fortune of being more efficient in the way they excrete uric acid. And children rarely get it.
Other risk factors include:

- **Middle age.** Men in their 40s and 50s are at greatest risk.
- **Family history of gout.** Up to 18 percent of all people with gout have family members with gout.
- **Overweight.** Excessive eating steps up the production of uric acid.
- Eating too many foods with purines, such as organ meats (liver, kidney, brains, sweetbreads), sardines, anchovies, meat extracts, dried peas, lentils, and legumes.
- An enzyme defect that prevents the breakdown of uric acid.
- Heavy alcohol use.
- Exposure to environmental lead.
- Using certain medications, including diuretics, salicylates, and levodopa.
- Taking niacin, a vitamin that's also called nicotinic acid.

Gout symptoms come on quickly the first time, often overnight. You can go to bed feeling fine and wake up later in excruciating pain. You may also experience joint swelling and shiny red or purple skin around the joint. **If you're already predisposed to gout, you can trigger an episode by**

- Drinking too much alcohol
- Overeating, especially purine foods
- Having surgery
- Experiencing a sudden severe illness or trauma
- Going on a crash diet

- Injuring a joint
- Having chemotherapy
- Being under stress. The link isn't the stress itself, but the comfort eating or drinking that may accompany it.

If you have gout, professional medical treatment is required. There are several prescription medications that are very effective at eliminating excess uric acid. Untreated, gout may progress to serious joint damage and disability. Also, excess uric acid can cause kidney stones. For gout, though, there are several kitchen remedies that can be effective along with medication to alleviate the pain and symptoms.

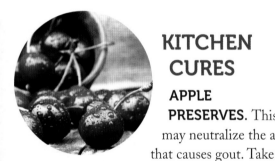

KITCHEN CURES

APPLE PRESERVES. This may neutralize the acid that causes gout. Take as many apples as you wish, then peel, core, and slice. Simmer in a little water for three hours or more, until they turn thick, brown, and sweet. Refrigerate. Use as you would any preserve.

CELERY SEED. It neutralizes acid in the body, including the uric acid that builds up to cause gout. Crush 1 to 2 teaspoons celery seeds and place in a cup of boiling water. Steep 20 minutes, strain, then sweeten to cover the bitter taste. Drink 1 cup three times a day.

CHERRIES. Cherries may remove toxins from the body, clean the kidneys, and yes, even help give you a rosy complexion. Because of their cleansing power, they're at the top of the gout-relief list. If you can bake a cherry pie, you may be making a gout treatment. Cherry compote, cherry juice, cherry jam, cherry tea, cherry anything works.

CHICORY. If you've been to New Orleans, you know the flavor. It's in the coffee, and it's definitely an acquired taste. Chicory is an old herb, its first use recorded around the first century A.D., and over the past 2,000 years it's seen many medicinal uses. Gout is one of them. Here's a recipe said to relieve symptoms. Mix 1 ounce chicory root to 1 pint boiling water, and take as much of it as you want. This can work as a poultice, too, when it is applied to the skin in the area affected by gout.

FIGS. Crush and boil 4 figs in 1 pint water. Cook until half the water is gone. Cool, then drink.

THYME. Drink as a tea. Add 1 to 2 teaspoons to a cup of boiling water. Sweeten, and drink.

WATER. To rid yourself of uric acid, you absolutely must keep your body flushed out.

Drink at least 2 quarts of water a day—more, if you can manage it.

MORE DO'S & DON'TS

- Take fish oil supplements to ease the inflammation that comes with gout.

- Avoid turkey meat, organ meats, herring, anchovies, meat gravies, beer, and red wine. These are high in purines, which are metabolized to uric acid.

GOOD FOODS, BAD FOODS

Diet plays an important role in gout prevention. **Here are some foods that will help to keep gout under control:**

Whole-grain cereals and whole-wheat bread. These are loaded with zinc that may be depleted during a gout attack.

Breakfast cereals and breads fortified with folic acid. These can slow the production of uric acid.

Bread, pasta, low fat milk and dairy products, eggs, lettuce, tomatoes. These are low-purine foods.

Citrus fruits. They have vitamin C that may assist the kidneys in ridding the body of uric acid.

And if you have gout and don't want it to come back, avoid these foods:

Asparagus, spinach, cauliflower, mushrooms. They have purines.

Shrimp and crabs. They also contain purines.

Alcohol. It increases uric acid production in foods. That means beer, too!

Dried fruit and fruit sugar. If you eat it, do so in moderation. The fructose in it produces uric acid.

HANGOVERS

Well, you partied from sundown to sunup, and now you're paying the price. You've got the pounding headache, the queasiness, the dizziness, the sensitivity to light and sound, the muscle aches, and the irritability that comes from overconsumption of alcoholic beverages. How quickly last night's fun turns into next morning's nightmare when you have a hangover!

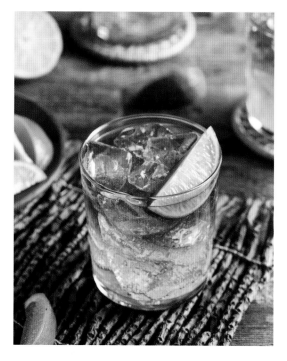

WHY SUCH SUFFERING?

Although we don't like to think of it as such, especially when we're having such a good time, alcohol is actually a drug. It's a depressant, and when taken in excess, it fills your body with toxins. Your body reacts as it would to any drug overdose: It tries to metabolize and get rid of the offending substances.

Researchers aren't sure what in the alcohol causes a hangover. But they do know that the debilitating symptoms you experience are a result of the body's inability to get rid of the toxins quickly enough, and they build up in your bloodstream.

Your body's attempts to flush out the alcohol puts a strain on the liver, which madly draws on the body's water reserves to get the job done. Since alcohol is a major diuretic, causing you to urinate more frequently, you lose more water than your body takes in with the beverage. As strange as it may sound, the more alcohol you drink, the more vital fluids you lose. The considerable water loss associated with drinking alcohol increases the liver's burden to get a hold of water anywhere it can. It will take water from the brain and from other vital organs. The resulting dehydration is what's behind many of the worst symptoms of a hangover.

The process of metabolizing the alcohol and excreting large quantities of water also robs the body of glucose and other vital nutrients. Being malnourished further contributes to the unpleasant hangover symptoms.

In addition to dehydration, fatigue is also behind some of your hangover pain. Excessive drinking and late nights usually go hand-in-hand. But more than that, alcohol interferes with a normal sleep pattern, robbing you of the dream state, which is essential to feeling rested. You may pass out on the floor and sleep for hours, but it won't be the kind of sleep that will allow you to restart your engines in the morning. Lack of proper rest contributes to the malaise a hangover brings.

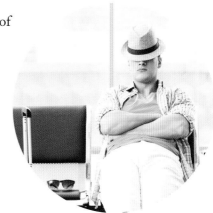

PREVENTION

The best way to prevent a hangover is, of course, drinking in moderation or abstaining from alcohol. But keeping yourself well-hydrated and well-nourished when you're drinking can go a long way toward minimizing the morning-after symptoms. Try drinking a glass of water or other noncaffeinated beverage for each alcoholic beverage you drink. And don't drink on an empty stomach. Food helps slow the absorption of alcohol, giving your body time to metabolize it and decreasing the chances of a hangover.

The best cure for a hangover: time. Of course, people ignore the prevention and don't have "time" for the cure. So, here are some remedies to ease the suffering for those who have had one drink too many.

KITCHEN CURES

BANANA. Bananas are your best friend! While you were drunk and peeing like a racehorse, lots of potassium drained from your body. Eating a banana bursting with potassium will give you some giddy-up and go. All you have to do is peel and eat.

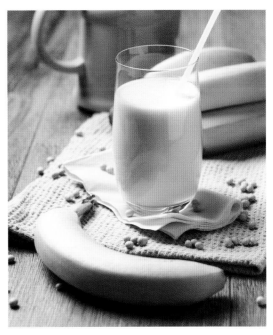

GINGER ROOT. Ginger has long been used to treat nausea and seasickness. And, since having a hangover is much like being seasick, this easy remedy works wonders. If you're really green, the best bet is to drink ginger ale (no preparation required). If you can remain vertical for ten minutes, brew some ginger

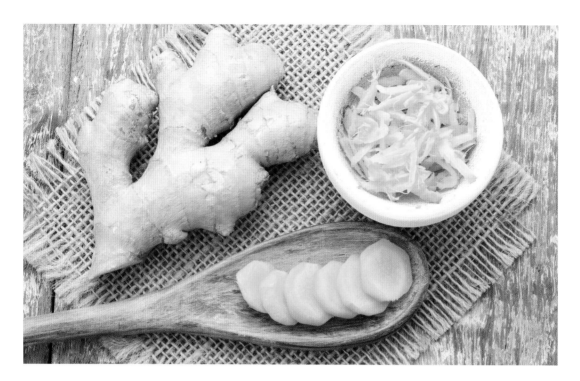

tea. Cut 10 to 12 slices of fresh ginger root and combine with 4 cups water. Boil for ten minutes. Strain and add the juice of 1 orange, the juice of ¹/₂ lemon, and ¹/₂ cup honey. Drink to your relief.

HONEY AND LEMON. The classic hot toddy (nonalcoholic, of course) is honey, lemon, and hot water. Easy to swallow, this beverage replenishes fluids and sugars lost to a hangover. It is vital, however, to use honey instead of white sugar. Honey contains fructose, which competes for the metabolism of alcohol. Some healthy competition is needed, since it prevents the rapid change in alcohol levels that results in headaches. Plain sugar contains sucrose, which isn't absorbed as quickly. To make a toddy, boil 1 cup water and mix in honey and lemon juice to taste. Enjoy a toddy several times a day.

JUICE. Juice, especially freshly squeezed orange juice, will help raise your blood sugar levels and help ease some of your hangover symptoms. However, if your stomach is upset, skip acidic juices such as orange juice and stick with apple juice instead.

RICE, SOUP, OR TOAST. Food is probably the last thing you want to look at while recovering, but you do need some substance for energy. Stay with clear liquids until you can tolerate something solid. Then start off slowly with mild, easy-to-digest foods such as plain toast, rice, or clear soup.

SPORTS DRINKS. These are a good way to replace fluids as well as electrolytes and glucose.

HANGOVER CURE MYTHS

Myth #1: A strong cuppa joe cures a hangover.

If only it were as easy as stopping off at Starbucks! Coffee does little, if anything, to help you sober up and may, in fact, work against you. Like alcohol, coffee is a diuretic and can further dehydrate your system. Moreover, the acidic nature of coffee can sour a sensitive stomach. What coffee can do is ease your aching headache by constricting blood vessels, but it does so at a price. Instead of brewing a cuppa, it's a better (and easier) idea to take two nonaspirin pain relievers, especially acetaminophen. Aspirin can aggravate the stomach.

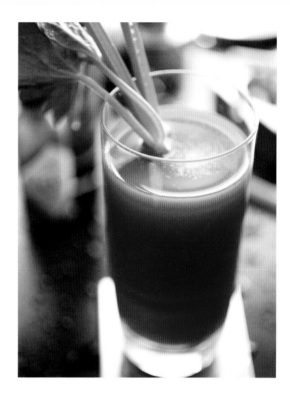

Myth #2: Slurp a raw egg and sober up.

You really have to be drunk to handle this unappetizing cure. Besides the strong possibility of vomiting, you risk salmonella poisoning if you down an uncooked egg. Another cure, equally repulsive, is the Prairie Oyster concoction: 1 egg yolk, a dash of Worcestershire sauce, a dash of ketchup, $1/2$ ounce port, a celery stick, salt and pepper. That's one drink that makes even the sober shudder.

Myth #3: A morning-after drink will cure a hangover.

Along the lines of the "hair-of-the-dog-that-bit-you" philosophy, drinking a glass of what you drank the night before (or any other alcohol for that matter) won't help. A morning-after drink only recreates the problem and worsens symptoms.

Myth #4: Down a big, all-American breakfast for a quick cure.

Greasy bacon, runny eggs, and fried potatoes will send you running to the toilet faster than you can say "hangover cure." The poor stomach, already irritated by alcohol, isn't prepared for this hard-to-digest, fatty trio. Give the tummy a break and stick to toast, perhaps with a little marmalade on top.

HEARTBURN

Boy, oh boy, did you do it this time. You added that heaping second helping to all the platter pickings you couldn't resist, and what do you have? Indigestion (an incomplete or imperfect digestion), that's what. And it may be accompanied by pain, nausea, vomiting, heartburn, gas, and belching. All this because you couldn't resist temptation. But don't worry. It happens to everybody, and it goes away.

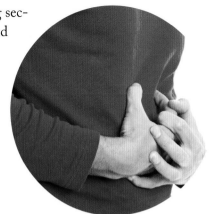

So, now that you've eaten until you're about ready to burst, what's next? The couch, maybe? Stretch out, let your digestive system do its thing, take a nap?

Wrong! The worst thing you can do after a binge is to lie down. That can cause heartburn, also known as acid indigestion. Whatever you call it, it's the feeling you get when digestive acid escapes your stomach and irritates the esophagus, the tube that leads from your throat to your stomach. After you eat, heartburn can also fire up when you:

- Bend forward
- Exercise
- Strain muscles

WHY ACID BACKS UP

Occasionally the acid keeps on coming until you have a mouthful of something bitter and acidy. You may have some pain in your gut, too, or in your chest. Along with that acid may come a belch, one that may bring even more of that stomach acid with it.

The purpose of stomach acid is to break down the foods we eat so our body can digest them. Our stomachs have a protective lining that shields it from those acids, but the esophagus does not have that protection. Normally that's not a problem, because after we swallow food, it passes down the esophagus, through a sphincter, and into the stomach. The sphincter then closes.

Occasionally, though, the muscles of that sphincter are weakened and it doesn't close properly or it doesn't close all the way. Scarring from an ulcer or frequent episodes of acid reflux (when the acid comes back up), stomach pressure from overeating, obesity, and pregnancy can all cause this glitch in the lower esophageal sphincter (LES). And when the LES gets a glitch and allows the gastric acid to splash out of the stomach, you get heartburn.

Generally, heartburn isn't serious. In fact, small amounts of reflux are normal and most people don't even notice it because the swallowing we do causes saliva to wash the acids right back down into the stomach where they belong. When the stomach starts shooting back amounts that are larger than normal, especially on a regular basis or over a prolonged period of time, that's when the real trouble begins, and simple heartburn can turn into esophageal inflammation or bleeding. Who's prone to heartburn? Just about anybody. According to the National Digestive Diseases Clearinghouse, 25 million adults suffer from heartburn daily and about 60 million Americans get gastroesophageal reflux and heartburn at least once a month.

There are several prescription medicines available for the treatment of long-term or serious heartburn or acid reflux, and over-the-counter remedies are available at your pharmacy, too. But there are several remedies right in your own kitchen that can fight the fire of heartburn.

FROM THE DRAWER

If you're prone to heartburn, keep a food diary. This can tell you which foods or food combinations cause that heartburn.

KITCHEN CURES

ALMONDS. Chewing 6 or 8 blanched almonds during an episode of heartburn may relieve the symptoms. Chew them well, though, to avoid swallowing air and causing yourself more discomfort.

APPLES. They cool the burn of stomach acid. Eat them fresh, with the skin still on, or cook them for desserts.

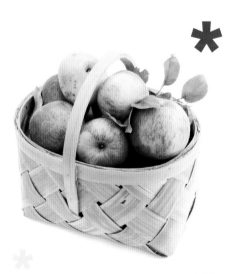

APPLE HONEY. This is a simple remedy that will neutralize stomach acids. Peel, core, and slice several sweet apples. Simmer with a little water over low heat for three hours until the mixture is thick, brown, and sweet to the taste. Refrigerate in an airtight container and take a few spoonfuls whenever you have the need.

BROWN RICE. Plain or with a little sweetening, rice can help relieve discomfort. Rice is a complex carbohydrate and is a bland food, which is less likely to increase acidity or relax the sphincter muscle

BUTTERMILK. This is an acid-reliever, but don't confuse it with regular milk, which can be an acid-maker, especially if you are bothered by lactose intolerance.

CABBAGE. Like apples, this is a natural fire extinguisher for stomach burn. For the best relief, put the cabbage through a juicer, then drink it.

CARDAMOM. This old-time digestive aid may help relieve the burn of acid indigestion. Add it to baked goodies such as sweet rolls or fruit cake, or sprinkle, with a pinch of cinnamon, on toast. It works well in cooked cereals, too.

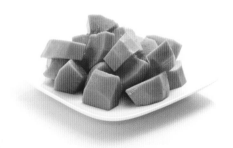

CINNAMON. This is a traditional remedy for acid relief. Brew a cup of cinnamon tea from a cinnamon stick. Or try a commercial brand, but check the label. Cinnamon tea often has black tea in it, which is a cause of heartburn, so make sure your commercial brand doesn't contain black tea. For another acid-busting treat, make cinnamon toast.

FRUIT JUICES. Skip juices from citrus fruits, but try these stomach-cooling juices for heartburn relief: papaya, mango, guava, pear.

GINGER. A tea from this root can soothe that burning belly. Add 1 ½ teaspoons ginger root to 1 cup water; simmer for ten minutes. Drink as needed.

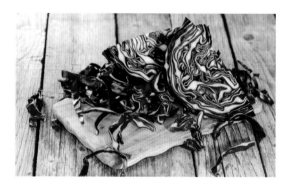

LIME JUICE. Mix 10 drops lime juice with ½ teaspoon sugar and ¼ teaspoon baking soda, in that order. When the baking soda is added it will fizz, and that's when you need to drink it down. The fizz will neutralize stomach acid.

PAPAYA. Eat it straight to reap the benefit of its natural, indigestion-fighting enzyme papain. Or drink 1 cup papaya juice combined with 1 teaspoon sugar and 2 pinches cardamom to relieve acid.

Warning! Pregnant women should not eat papayas; they're a source of natural estrogen that can cause miscarriage.

POTATO. Mix ½ cup raw potato juice with ½ cup water, and drink after meals. To make raw potato juice, simply put a peeled raw potato through a juicer or blender.

PUMPKIN. Eat it baked as a squash to get rid of heartburn. Fresh is best. Spice it up with cinnamon, which is another heartburn cure. Or, make a compote of baked pumpkin and apples, spiced with cinnamon and honey, for a dessert that's both curative and tasty.

SAGE. Use it to make a tea that can relieve stomach weakness that allows acid to be released back into the esophagus.

SODA CRACKERS. This is an old folk cure that actually works. Soda crackers (preferably unsalted) are bland, they digest easily, and they absorb stomach acid. They also contain bicarbonate of soda and cream of tartar, which neutralize the acid. **Tip:** You know that package of soda crackers they always give you at the restaurant, that you leave on the table? From now on, take them with you. These come in handy when you're plagued by heartburn and can't seek immediate relief.

YOGURT. Make sure it has live cultures in it. Because of the helpful and digestive-friendly microorganisms in yogurt, it may sooth the acid-forming imbalances that can lead to heartburn.

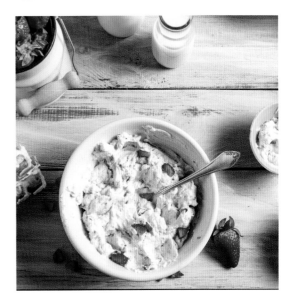

FIRE-FIGHTING FOODS

Proteins may strengthen the sphincter that allows the stomach acid to escape. Make sure all your meals contain some protein in order to keep that valve in good working order. **These top the sphincter-friendly list:**

- Lean meats
- Fish
- Poultry
- Low fat dairy products

MORE DO'S & DON'TS

- Eat smaller meals. The more food in your belly, the more likely that bulk will push stomach acid right back up.

- Eat slowly and chew thoroughly. Sometimes heartburn will flare because the food is simply too large to get through the digestive tract and it, along with the acids, is forced back up.

- Don't eat right before bedtime. Give your stomach a two- or three-hour break before you sleep.

THE USUAL SUSPECTS

Here's the food list that's commonly associated with heartburn. Cut back on these, or cut them out altogether, and see what happens:

Fried and fatty foods, pies, cakes, cookies, butter, margarine, oils, cream: These may weaken your LES. Also, fatty foods take longer to digest, meaning the gastric juices are working overtime and have more opportunity to cause a backup.

Peppermint in any form*: It relaxes the stomach muscle and valve, allowing the release of acids back up into the esophagus.

Caffeinated beverages, such as coffee, tea, cola: Caffeine causes extra acid production.

Chocolate: It contains methylxanthines, a second cousin to caffeine, and can weaken the stomach valve.

Fruit and vegetable juices, especially tomato and citrus juice: They can irritate the throat and cause pain if heartburn has already caused irritation. Pineapple juice has an especially potent punch.

Garlic and onions: May weaken the LES.

Spicy, pickled, or fermented foods: These are heartburn-makers, too.

Alcohol: It causes the LES to relax.

Smoking and certain drugs such as aspirin, ibuprofen, and some antibiotics: These also relax the LES, causing acid reflux.

*Warning! Peppermint is often prescribed for other symptoms of indigestion but should never be used when heartburn is present.

HEART DISEASE

The heart is an amazing structure, tough yet fragile. A muscle, its network of arteries and veins transport blood through your body, nourishing organs and tissues. When the heart is working as it should, you barely notice it. But when your heart starts acting strangely, you have cause to worry. Thankfully, you live in a day when heart disease can be treated very successfully, and in some cases, the condition can even be reversed.

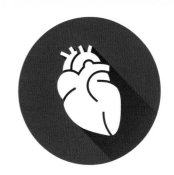

HEART TROUBLE

Heart disease is any condition that keeps your heart from functioning at its best or causes a deterioration of the heart's arteries and vessels. Coronary heart disease (CHD), also known as coronary artery disease, is the most common form of heart disease, affecting 12.6 million people in America. If you are diagnosed with CHD, it means you have atherosclerosis, or hardening of the arteries on the heart's surface. Arteries become hard when plaque accumulates on artery walls. This plaque develops gradually as an overabundance of low-density lipoprotein (LDL) cholesterol (the bad stuff) makes itself at home in your arteries. The plaque builds and narrows the artery walls, making it more and more difficult for blood to pass through the heart and increasing the opportunity for a blood clot to form. If the heart doesn't get enough blood, it can cause chest pain (angina) or a heart attack.

Not treating coronary heart disease can also lead to congestive heart failure (CHF). CHF happens when your heart isn't strong enough to pump blood throughout the body—it fails to meet the body's need for oxygen. This often causes congestion in the lungs and a variety of other problems for your heart and the rest of your body.

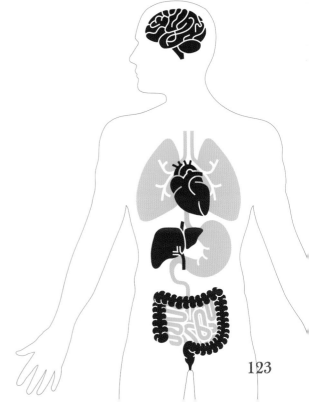

HONING IN ON HEART DISEASE

There are many risk factors for heart disease, some you can do something about, and some you can't. A family history of heart disease puts you at much greater risk for developing it yourself. While you can't do anything about your genes, there are a number of risk factors that you can control. **These are the ones you can do something about:**

- High levels of low-density lipoprotein (LDL) cholesterol (the bad stuff), and low levels of high-density lipoprotein (the good stuff).
- High levels of triglycerides. Triglyceride levels increase when you eat too many fatty foods or when you eat too much—excess calories are made into triglycerides and stored as fat in cells. Having an abundance of triglycerides has been linked to coronary heart disease.

- High blood pressure
- Smoking
- Lack of regular exercise
- A high fat diet
- Being overweight or obese
- Diabetes
- Ongoing stress or depression

Your best strategies for fighting heart disease will be developed by you and your medical team. But you can find help in food as well.

KITCHEN CURES

BRAN. Bran cereal is a high-fiber food that will help keep your cholesterol levels in check. Other high fiber foods in your cupboard include barley, oats, whole grains such as brown rice and lentils, and beans, such as kidney beans and black beans.

BROCCOLI. Calcium is another heart-healthy nutrient, and milk isn't the only calcium-rich food. In fact, there are lots of nondairy foods that are rich in calcium, such as kale, salmon, figs, pinto beans, and okra. One cup of broccoli can supply you with 90 mg of calcium.

CHICKEN. Three ounces of chicken will give you $1/3$ of your daily requirement for vitamin B6, a necessary nutrient for maintaining heart health.

GARLIC. Chock full of antioxidants, garlic seems to be able to lessen plaque buildup, reduce the incidence of chest pain, and keep the heart generally healthy. It is also a mild anticoagulant, helping to thin the blood. The advantages may take some time: One study found that it took a couple of years of eating garlic daily to get its heart-healthy benefits.

OLIVE OIL. The American Heart Association and the American Dietetic Association recommend getting most of your fat from monounsaturated sources. Olive oil is a prime candidate. Try using it instead of other vegetable oils when sautéing your veggies.

PEANUT BUTTER. Eat 2 tablespoons of this comforting food and you can get $^1/_3$ of your daily intake of vitamin E. Because vitamin E is a fat-soluble vitamin (other antioxidant vitamins are water soluble), it is found more abundantly in fattier foods like vegetable oils and nuts. If you're watching your weight, don't go overboard on the peanut butter.

PECANS. These tasty nuts are full of magnesium, another heart-friendly nutrient. One ounce of pecans drizzled over a spinach salad can give you $^1/_3$ of your recommended daily allowance of this vital mineral.

SALMON. Adding fatty fish to your diet is a good idea if you're at risk for heart disease. Three ounces of salmon meets your daily requirement for vitamin B12, a vitamin that helps keep your heart healthy, and it's a good source of omega-3 fatty acids, which have been proven to lower triglycerides and reduce blood clots that could potentially block arteries in the heart.

SPINACH. Make yourself a salad using spinach instead of the usual iceberg lettuce and get a good start on meeting your folic acid needs ($^1/_2$ cup has 130 mcg of folic acid). Along with the other B vitamins, B6 and B12, folic acid can help prevent heart disease.

STRAWBERRIES. Oranges aren't the only fruit loaded with vitamin C. You can fill up on 45 milligrams of the heart healthy vitamin with $^1/_2$ cup of summer's sweet berry. Vitamin C is an antioxidant vital to maintaining a happy heart. Strawberries are also a good source of fiber and potassium, both important to heart health.

SWEET POTATOES. With double your daily requirements for vitamin A, a heart-protecting nutrient, sweet potatoes are a smart choice for fending off heart disease.

WHOLE-WHEAT BREAD. Slather some peanut butter on a slice of whole-wheat bread and you've got a snack that's good to your heart. One slice of whole-wheat bread has 11 mcg of selenium, an antioxidant mineral that works with vitamin E to protect your heart.

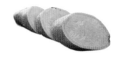

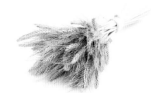

HOW WHAT YOU EAT AFFECTS YOUR HEART

Scientists have been looking at the link between food and your heart for decades, and while research is still ongoing, there is one definite conclusion: What you put in your body can help, or hurt, your heart. Recent research discovered that there are some specific nutrients that do indeed help keep your heart healthy and can even reverse the effects of heart disease.

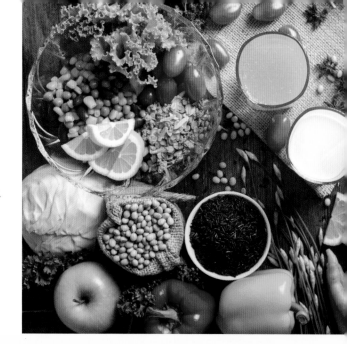

ANTIOXIDANTS

Sources: Vitamins A, C, and E and selenium
What they do: A couple of things. First, they keep LDL cholesterol (the bad cholesterol) from oxidizing; that's why they're called antioxidants. Preventing the oxidation process keeps plaque from building up in the arteries. These valuable nutrients also block oxygen-free radicals (another reason for the name) that can cause plaque buildup in the arteries. Bottom line: They reduce the risk of atherosclerosis, or hardening of the arteries, which can lead to heart disease, heart attack, and stroke.

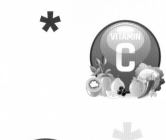

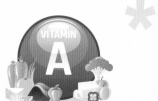

How much you need:

- **Vitamin A:** After age 11, men need 900 REs a day; women need 700 REs a day (RE is retinol equivalent—it's the way scientists measure amounts of the vitamin).

- **Vitamin C:** Adult men need 90 mg a day, while adult women need 75.

- **Vitamin E:** Adults need 15 mg a day.

- **Selenium:** Adults need 55 micrograms (mcg) per day.

B VITAMINS

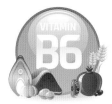

Sources: Vitamins B6, B12, and folic acid

What they do: When your body digests meat, it raises the homocysteine levels in your blood. When you have high levels of homocysteine, you're more at risk for clogged arteries and blood clots. Eating a sufficient amount of B vitamins can help turn homocysteine into something harmless to your body, lessening your chances of developing plaque in your arteries.

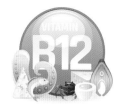

How much you need:

- **Vitamin B6:** Up to age 50 you need 1.3 mg a day; after 50 men's needs rise to 1.7 mg a day, while women over 50 need 1.5 mg daily.

- **Vitamin B12:** All adults need 2.4 mcg a day.

- **Folic Acid:** Men and women older than 14 need 400 mcg daily.

MINERALS

Sources: Calcium and magnesium

What they do: Calcium reduces the risk of death from heart disease, lowers blood pressure, and lowers cholesterol. Magnesium is vital to keeping your heart healthy. It helps prevent plaque buildup and strengthens artery walls. And if you have a heart attack, having adequate amounts of magnesium in your body can increase your chances of surviving.

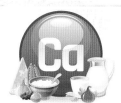

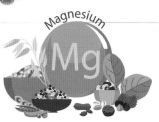

How much you need:

- **Calcium:** Adults up to age 50 need 1,000 mg a day. After 50 women's calcium needs rise a bit to 1,200 mg daily, and after age 70 everyone should be getting 1,200 mg daily.

- **Magnesium:** From 19 to 30, men need 400 mg a day. After age 30, men need 420 mg. From ages 19 to 30, women need 310 mg; they need 320 mg daily after age 30.

HIGH BLOOD PRESSURE

Sometimes what you don't know can hurt you. Such is the case with high blood pressure, or hypertension. Although one in four adults has high blood pressure, according to the American Heart Association (AHA), almost a third of them don't know they have it.

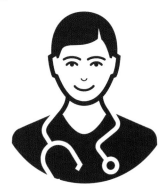

That's because high blood pressure often has no symptoms. It's not as if you feel the pressure of your blood coursing through your circulatory system. When the heart beats, it pumps blood to the arteries, creating pressure within them. That pressure can be normal or it can be excessive. High blood pressure is defined as a persistently elevated pressure of blood within the arteries.

Over time, the excessive force exerted against the arteries damages and scars them. It can also damage organs, such as the heart, kidneys, and brain. High blood pressure can lead to strokes, blindness, kidney failure, and heart failure.

In 90 to 95 percent of all cases, the cause of high blood pressure isn't known. In such cases, when there is no underlying cause, the disease is known as primary, or essential, hypertension. Sometimes the high blood pressure is caused by another disease, such as an endocrine disorder. In such cases the disease is called secondary hypertension.

The key to controlling high blood pressure is knowing you have it. Under the guidance of a physician, you can battle hypertension through diet, exercise, lifestyle changes, and medication, if necessary. The kitchen holds several blood pressure helpers.

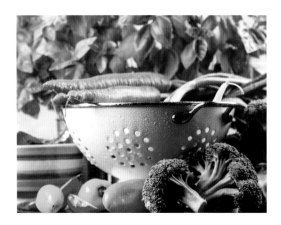

EATING FRESH

If you have high blood pressure or are at risk for it, skip processed foods. Not only are they loaded with sodium (salt) but they are also high in saturated (read: artery-clogging) fat. Read labels, as it's not always obvious which foods contain the most sodium and saturated fat.

KITCHEN CURES

BANANAS. The banana has been proved to help reduce blood pressure. The average person needs three to four servings of potassium-rich fruits and vegetables each day. Some experts believe doubling this amount may benefit your blood pressure. If bananas aren't your favorite bunch of fruit, try dried apricots, raisins, currants, orange juice, spinach, boiled potatoes with skin, baked sweet potatoes, cantaloupe, and winter squash.

BREADS. Be good to your blood with a bit more "B," as in the B vitamin folate. Swimming around the blood is a substance called homocysteine, which at high levels is thought to reduce the stretching ability of the arteries. If the arteries are stiff as a board, the heart pumps extra hard to move the blood around. Folate helps reduce the levels of homocysteine, in turn helping arteries become pliable. You'll find folate in fortified breads and cereals, asparagus, Brussels sprouts, and beans.

BROCCOLI. This vegetable is high in fiber, and a high fiber diet is known to help reduce blood pressure. So indulge in this and other fruits and vegetables that are high in fiber.

CANOLA, MUSTARD SEED, OR SAF-FLOWER OILS. Switching to polyunsaturated oils can make a big difference in your blood pressure readings. Switching to them will also reduce your blood cholesterol level.

CAYENNE PEPPER. This fiery spice is a popular home treatment for mild high blood pressure. Cayenne pepper allows smooth blood flow by preventing platelets from clumping together and accumulating in the blood. Add some cayenne pepper to salt-free seasonings, or add a dash to a salad or in salt-free soups.

CELERY. Because it contains high levels of 3-N-butylphthalide, a phytochemical that helps lower blood pressure, celery is in a class by itself. This phytochemical is not found in most other vegetables. Celery may also reduce stress hormones that constrict blood vessels, so it may be most effective in those whose high blood pressure is the result of mental stress.

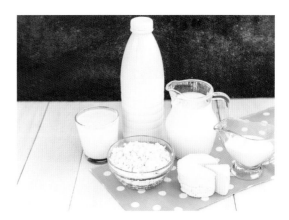

MILK. The calcium in milk does more than build strong bones; it plays a modest role in preventing high blood pressure. Be sure to drink skim milk or eat low fat yogurt. Leafy green vegetables also provide calcium.

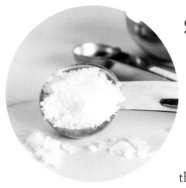

SALT WEARS MANY DISGUISES

Lose the saltshaker. Although there is some debate about salt's role in high blood pressure, most experts agree that cutting back on salt intake can reduce blood pressure. Sodium chloride isn't the only name for salt. Soda or sodium also indicate the presence of salt. Look closely at labels for these sources of salt.

- Monosodium glutamate (MSG) is a popular flavor enhancer in restaurant cooking and in packaged and canned foods and seasoning mixes.

- Baking soda (sodium bicarbonate or bicarbonate of soda) and baking power are often used to leaven breads and cakes.

- Disodium phosphate is found in some quick-cooking cereals and processed cheeses.

- Sodium alginate is what makes ice cream smooth.

- Sodium benzoate is used as a preservative in many condiments.

- Sodium hydroxide is used to soften and loosen skins of ripe olives and certain fruits and vegetables.

- Sodium nitrate is used to cure meats and sausages.

- Sodium propionate helps inhibit the growth of molds in baked goods.

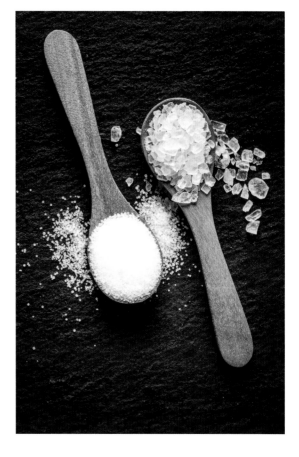

- Sodium sulfite is used to bleach foods that will then be colored or glazed. It's also used as a preservative in some dried fruits.

HIGH CHOLESTEROL

Cholesterol is that waxy, soft stuff that floats around in your bloodstream as well as in all the cells in your body. It takes a bad rap these days because the word cholesterol strikes fear in the hearts of even the healthiest of people.

Having cholesterol in your blood is normal and even healthy because it's used in the formation of cell membranes, tissues, and essential hormones. So, in proper amounts, cholesterol is good. In excessive amounts, though, it can clog the arteries leading to your heart and cause coronary disease, heart attack, or stroke.

Cholesterol comes from two sources: the foods you eat and your very own liver. And the truth of the matter is, your liver can produce all the cholesterol your body will ever need. This means that what you get in your food isn't necessary. Some people get rid of extra cholesterol easily through normal bodily waste mechanisms, but others hang on to it because their bodies just aren't as efficient in removing it, which puts them at risk.

So, what makes people prone to high blood cholesterol?

- Family history
- Eating too many foods high in saturated fats
- Diabetes
- Kidney and liver disorders
- Alcoholism
- Obesity
- Smoking
- Stress

GOOD AND BAD CHOLESTEROL?

There are two different kinds of cholesterol, and yes, one's good and one's bad. Cholesterol can't get around on its own, so it hitches a ride from lipoproteins to get to the body's cells. Problem is, there are two different rigs picking it up: One is called HDL, or high-density lipoprotein, the other is called LDL, or low-density lipoprotein. HDL is the good ride; it travels away from your arteries. LDL is the bad ride; it heads straight to your arteries. **Bottom line: HDL is what you want more of; you want less of LDL.**

High cholesterol can be cured two ways: by medication and/or by diet. There are numerous effective drugs on the market that will make drastic reductions in cholesterol levels, but they all come with side effects and require frequent blood tests to monitor for possible problems. But there are kitchen cures, and they may work on their own or along with conventional treatment. Whatever your cure, it must come with advice from your doctor since your heart is at risk.

KITCHEN CURES

ALFALFA SPROUTS. These may improve or normalize cholesterol levels.
Warning! Sprouts are not clean or washed when you buy them in the store, and they may be a source of *E.coli* bacteria. Wash thoroughly before you consume or use a veggie-cleaning product available in most grocery stores.

ALMONDS. Studies indicate that snacking on almonds regularly for as little as three weeks may decrease LDL by up to ten percent.

APPLES. Apples are high in pectin, which can lower cholesterol levels.

ARTICHOKES. This veggie can actually lower cholesterol levels. Early studies pointed to their beneficial cholesterol-busting properties, but more recent studies have shown that artichokes may be even more effective than they were first thought to be.

BEETS. Full of carotenoids and flavonoids, beets help lower—and may even prevent—the formation of LDL, the bad cholesterol.

CARROTS. Full of pectin, they're as good as apples in lowering cholesterol levels.

GARLIC. Studies show that garlic may not only reduce LDL but raise HDL and decrease the amount of fat in your blood. Add some fresh garlic regularly to your cooking to keep your heart healthy.

HONEY. Add 1 teaspoon honey to 1 cup hot water in the morning, and you may rid your system of excess fat and cholesterol, according to Ayurvedic medicine. Add 1 teaspoon lime juice or 10 drops cider vinegar to give that drink a more powerful cholesterol-fighting punch.

OATS. In any pure form, oats are a traditional cholesterol buster. Eating only ½ cup oatmeal a day, along with a low fat diet, may reduce cholesterol levels by nine percent.

OLIVE OIL. It protects your heart by lowering LDL, raising HDL, and preventing your blood from forming clots.

PEARS. These are high in soluble fiber, which helps regulate cholesterol levels.

RHUBARB. Yep, this is a cholesterol-buster. Consume it after a meal that's heavy in fats. You can cook it in a double boiler, with a little honey or maple syrup for added sweetness, until done. Add cardamom or vanilla if you like.

RICE. The oil that comes from the bran of rice is known to lower cholesterol. And brown rice is particularly high in fiber, which is essential in a cholesterol-lowering diet. One cup provides 11 percent of the daily fiber requirement.

SOYBEANS. These beauties may reduce LDL by as much as 20 percent when 25 to 50 grams of soy protein are eaten daily for as short a time as a month. Besides that obvious benefit, soy may fend off a rise in LDL in people with normal levels and also improve the ability of arteries to dilate. This means they expand better to allow the unimpeded passage of fats and other substances that otherwise might cause a blockage.

TURMERIC. This may lower blood cholesterol. Added to eggplant, you may reap twice the cholesterol-fighting benefit. Mix ³/₄ teaspoon turmeric with 2 tablespoons cooked, mashed eggplant and 1 ¹/₂ tablespoons boiling water. Spread it on whole wheat bread and eat after a meal heavy in fats.

WALNUTS. A cholesterol-lowering diet that includes walnuts eaten at least four times a week may lower LDL by as much as 16 percent. And studies indicate that those who munch on these nuts regularly cut their risk of death by heart attack in half when compared to non-walnut munchers.

YOGURT. Eating 1 cup plain yogurt with active cultures a day may reduce LDL by four percent or more and total cholesterol by at least three percent. Some scientists believe that eating yogurt regularly may even reduce the overall risk of heart disease by as much as ten percent.

FAT FACT

The more liquid the margarine (tub, liquid form), the less hydrogenated it is and the less trans fatty acid it contains. Trans fatty acids raise total blood cholesterol levels, so the less of them you eat, the better off you are.

MORE DO'S & DON'TS

- Don't grease those pans. Use a nonstick olive oil spray or buy an inexpensive oil mister in a kitchenwares store and make your own spray.

- Bulk up. Whole grains are high in fiber. Stick to complex carbohydrates, too, because they fill you up faster and leave you feeling satisfied. Try eating more fruits, veggies, pasta, rice.

- Read the food labels. They list the cholesterol content, so keep your cholesterol goal in mind: less than 300 mg a day.

- Eat small meals. Instead of 3 big meals a day, go for 5 or 6 small meals. The body deals with cholesterol intake more efficiently when it comes in small amounts.

INSOMNIA

The house is completely quiet. The kids are in bed. Your spouse is sawing logs. But you are staring at the ceiling listening to the fan hum. You've tried everything: counting sheep, counting dots on the ceiling, reading War and Peace, watching old sitcoms. But nothing is working. So you resign yourself to another dreary day of being a poster child for the walking dead.

Thirty to forty million Americans have some sort of trouble sleeping. There are more than 60 sleep disorders that plague men and women, from sleep apnea to restless legs syndrome. The number one sleep problem for men and women is insomnia. The National Sleep Foundation reports that 48 percent of Americans have insomnia occasionally, and 22 percent deal with sleeplessness almost every night. This wouldn't be such an unsettling statistic if lack of sleep was no big deal. But your body and mind need to shut down for a while at the end of the day.

INSUFFERABLE INSOMNIA

Insomnia can be classified in one of three ways—trouble falling asleep (called sleep-onset insomnia), trouble staying asleep (called sleep-maintenance insomnia), or waking up feeling groggy and sleepy after what should have been a full night's sleep. Most episodes of insomnia last anywhere from a couple of nights to a few weeks. There are myriad causes, including stress, anxiety, depression, disease, pain, medications, or simply not creating a relaxing sleep routine.

There's no magic number when it comes to how many hours you should sleep. Some people get by just fine on a few hours, and some people need more than eight. But it won't be a mystery to you if you're not getting enough sleep. Waking up exhausted and being sleepy most of the day are signs that you're not well-rested.

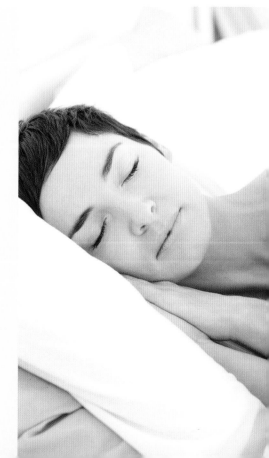

SUFFERING THROUGH
SLEEPLESS NIGHTS

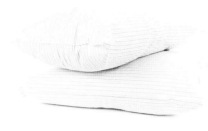

Women are 1.3 times more likely to experience insomnia than men. And if you're over age 65, you're 1.5 times more likely to have trouble sleeping than someone younger. Having problems in your marriage makes you more likely to have insomnia, as do hormonal changes such as those that occur during menopause, menstruation, and pregnancy.

INSOMNIA'S ILL EFFECTS

Insomnia can have a significant impact on your health and well-being. If you don't get enough sleep, you're setting yourself up for some serious problems. **People with insomnia are**

- Four times more likely to be diagnosed with depression.
- More likely to have a serious illness, including heart disease.
- More likely to have an accident on the job, at home, or on the road.
- More likely to miss work and accomplish less on the job than well-rested coworkers.

Fortunately, you can find some relief in food.

WHEN YOUR LEGS WANT TO DO
SOME WALKING...BUT YOU WANT TO SLEEP

Restless legs syndrome is a frustrating condition. The name of the problem explains it all. When you finally get into bed, your legs decide it's time to get up and move. The symptoms of restless legs syndrome have been described as tingling, crawling, or prickling sensations that peak during times of inactivity, such as when you're trying to go to sleep. Walking, massaging your legs, or taking a hot shower can help relieve the problem for a bit, but it'll come back, leaving you with a sleep-deprived night. Restless legs syndrome has been connected with a deficiency in iron and folic acid. The problem worsens with age and is more frequently diagnosed in people over 65. It can be treated with prescription medicines.

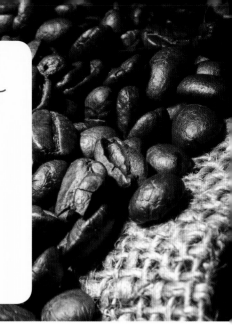

DRINKS TO AVOID 〰️

- Cut out the caffeine. Caffeine, by its nature, stimulates your brain. When you're trying to snooze, caffeine can cause problems. Having a couple of cups of coffee or a soda early in the day is fine, but switch to decaf after lunch.

- Avoid alcohol. Yes, alcohol is a sedative, but the effects soon wear off and you'll end up tossing and turning.

KITCHEN CURES

COOKIES. Yes, that comforting nighttime snack of milk and cookies may be just what the doctor ordered to get you back in bed. Sugary foods eaten about 30 minutes before bedtime can actually act as a sedative, and you can wake up without the morning fuzziness that accompanies synthetic sleeping pills. Be careful to eat only a few cookies, though; eating too much sugar can keep the sandman at bay.

DILL SEED. Though scientists haven't proved its worth, this herb is often used as a folk cure for insomnia in China. Its essential oil has the most sedative-producing properties.

HONEY. Folk remedies often advise people with sleeping difficulty to eat a little honey. It has the same sedative effect as sugar and may get you to bed more quickly. Try adding

1 tablespoon honey to some decaffeinated herbal tea or even to your warm milk for a relaxing pre-sleep drink.

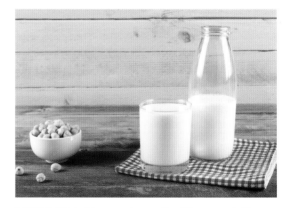

MILK. Drinking a glass of milk, especially a glass of warm milk, before bedtime is an age-old treatment for sleeping troubles. There is some debate, however, about what it is in milk—if anything—that helps cause slumber. Some scientists believe it's the presence of tryptophan, a chemical that helps the brain ease into sleep mode, that does the trick. Others believe it may be another ingredient, a soothing group of opiatelike chemicals called casomorphins. Whatever the reason, milk seems to help some people hit the sack more easily. And warm milk seems to be more effective at relaxing body and mind. Other foods high on the tryptophan scale are cottage cheese, cashews, chicken, turkey, soybeans, and tuna.

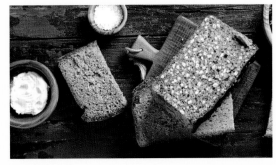

TOAST. High carbohydrate, low-protein bedtime snacks can make sleeping easier. Carbohydrate-rich foods tend to be easy on the tummy and can ease the brain into blissful slumber.

HERBS THAT HELP YOU SLEEP

Sleep problems have been around since biblical times, so it's no wonder that there are many, many botanical remedies for insomnia. Here are a few of the most common.

Chamomile. Chamomile tea is one of the most popular sleep-inducing drinks on the market. It's been used in folk medicine for years and is best used for sleep problems due to upset stomach. To brew your own chamomile tea: Put 1 heaping tablespoon chamomile flowers in a cup. Add boiling water, cover, and let steep for ten minutes.

Ginseng. Drinking a ginseng wine may help sleepless nights, especially if they're related to stress or a fever-producing illness. Chop 3 1/2 ounces ginseng (use only American ginseng) and place in 1 quart liquor, such as vodka. Let it stand for five to six weeks in a cool, dark place. Turn the container frequently. Take 1 ounce before bed.

FROM THE SUPPLEMENT ✳ SHELF

MELATONIN. Melatonin is the timekeeper of the body. It's a hormone that regulates your biological clock. As you get older you make less melatonin, which experts believe is probably why older folks have more trouble sleeping. Research is showing that taking a melatonin supplement can help you sleep. Ask your doctor about taking 1 to 3 mg of melatonin 1 1/2 to 2 hours before bedtime.

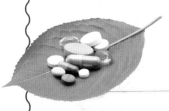

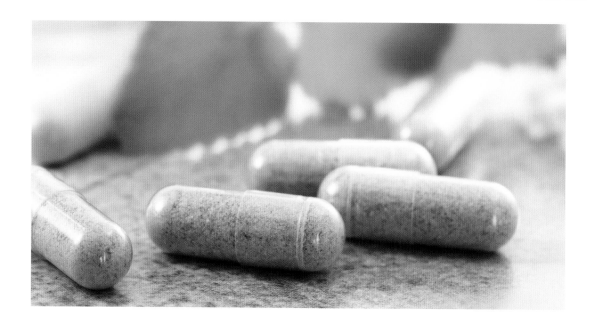

Lavender. The scent of lavender is so calming that in one study it was actually as potent as a tranquilizer. In Germany, where herbs are prescribed for medical conditions, doctors often give lavender for insomnia. You can find lavender essential oil at natural food stores.

Valerian. United States physicians listed this potent herb as a sedative until the late 19th century. Studies have found that it's as effective as Valium in coaxing sleep in some people, but it can act as a stimulant in others. Use cautiously. These days valerian is often combined with another herb, such as hops, to avoid any overstimulating effects.

Other herbs that might have a hand in getting you to catch some ZZZs are catnip, cinnamon, clove, hops, juniper, pine, passionflower, peppermint, sage, and skullcap. The best way to get the most relaxing effect from most of these herbs is to drink them in warm teas. Drink $1/2$ cup an hour before bedtime and a second dose right before you hit the sack.

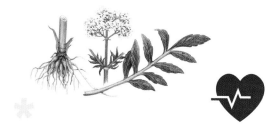

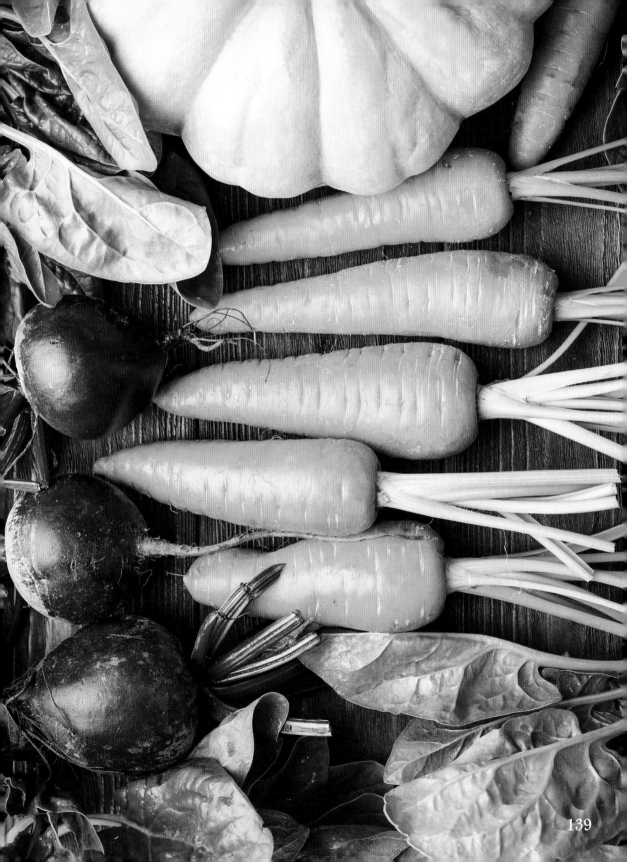

IRRITABLE BOWEL SYNDROME

Does this sound familiar? You're enjoying the evening, having a nice meal at a nice restaurant, feeling pretty good. Coffee and dessert come and you're lingering over pleasant conversation, then all of a sudden wham! Out of the blue you've got a belly cramp, a gut gurgle that registers a 3.5 on the Richter scale. And suddenly you're off to find the nearest facility. There was no warning, no nothing. It just hit, and now your evening is on hold, changed, or canceled until you see how this latest attack resolves itself.

Irritable Bowel Syndrome (IBS) is a real condition, with real symptoms. (A decade ago it was one of those things doctors thought was just "in your head.") But it's a mysterious one to medical experts, who still don't know what it is or what causes it exactly. What they do know is that it's common—about 15 percent of all adults are afflicted with it sometime in their lives—and that it is a malfunction of the digestive tract.

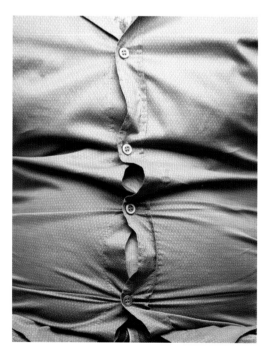

Symptoms of irritable bowl syndrome include

- Diarrhea or constipation, or alternate bouts of each
- Abdominal pain or cramping
- Gas and bloating
- Nausea, especially after eating
- Headache
- Fatigue
- Depression or anxiety
- Mucus-covered stools
- The urge to have another bowel movement after you've just had one

WHAT WE KNOW

Irritable bowel syndrome is also called spastic colon. It's an apt name that describes the abnormal digestive function that's typical of IBS. Normally, food is pushed through the intestine by synchronized muscle contractions. They are all dancing the same dance. But then something happens and one of those dancers steps out of the chorus line, does its own dance, and messes up everybody else's rhythm. As a result, the food that's being passed down that chorus line is suddenly disrupted in its travel.

Why does the muscle contraction become unsynchronized? No one knows for sure. Stress and poor diet are at the top of the suspected culprit list, since the majority of people with IBS seem either to be stressed-out or to have poor dietary habits. But that's only a guess. The other triggers most likely to cause it are: food intolerance, abdominal operations, medications, and hormonal changes during menstruation.

IBS is frustrating and inconvenient, but it's not serious, even though it does stand shoulder to shoulder with the common cold as a major reason for people to miss work. But the good news is, IBS doesn't lead to other more serious intestinal conditions. And it can be treated with medications that relieve the symptoms. However, treatment isn't always easy, since the cause isn't known. Regardless of the source of the problem, it does seem that there are some remedies for IBS symptoms right in your own kitchen.

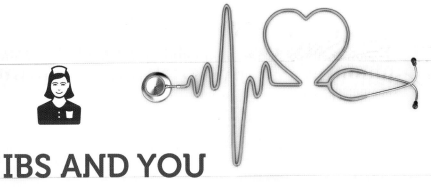

IBS AND YOU

Keep a food diary and track the foods that seem to trigger the attacks. Eliminate a specific food for a couple of weeks to see if that makes a difference. If it does, you may have isolated the cause. If not, go back to your food diary, then choose another food you've eaten around the time of an attack and eliminate it. This is called an exclusion diet, and if what you're eating is a trigger for IBS, this is the best way to find out what it is. Also make note of anxiety or stress you're feeling and what you think is causing it. If you notice that your attacks seem to come during stressful events, you may need to consider ways to eliminate them.

KITCHEN CURES

CABBAGE. Juice of the cabbage soothes the symptoms of intestinal ills. To turn this veggie into juice, simply wash and put through a juicer or blender. If these are not available to you, cook the cabbage in a very small amount of water—just enough to keep it from scorching or burning—until very mushy. Then pulverize with a fork or mixer.

CARROTS. These little gems help prevent the symptoms of IBS as well as regulate diarrhea and constipation. Eat them raw, by themselves or in salads, or eat them cooked—steamed and tossed with a little melted butter and brown sugar for a sweet treat. You can put raw carrots through the juicer, too. Since they're not a juicy veggie to begin with, add a little pure apricot nectar when you make carrot juice. Any way you eat a carrot is fine, just don't overcook them so much that you boil out all the goodness.

FENNEL SEEDS. These can relieve the intestinal spasms associated with IBS. They may also aid in the elimination of fats from the digestive system, inhibiting the over-production of mucus in the intestine, which is a symptom of the ailment. Steep the seeds into a tea by adding $1/2$ teaspoon fennel to 1 cup boiling water. Or add them to veggies such as carrots or cabbage, both of which soothe IBS symptoms. You can also sprinkle the seeds on salads or roast them and snack on them after a meal to reduce the symptoms of IBS and freshen your breath. To roast, spritz a baking sheet with olive oil, then cover with fennel seeds. Bake at 325°F for 10 to 15 minutes.

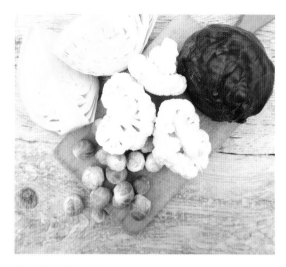

FLAXSEED. Make a tea using 1 teaspoon flaxseed per cup of water, and drink at bedtime for relief of symptoms.

LETTUCE. You can eat it raw to relieve symptoms of IBS, but it's especially helpful if lightly steamed. And when you're picking out your lettuce, go for the darker varieties. The darker the color, the more nutrients it contains.

OAT BRAN. Increasing fiber is a cure for almost every intestinal ill, and oat bran is especially good for IBS because it's mild and usually colon-friendly. So use some every day: a bowl of oatmeal, oat bran bread, oatmeal cookies. But don't expect immediate results. It may take up to a month to get any IBS relief.

PEARS. Fresh, ripe, sweet pears are a nutritious fruit that also helps relieve the symptoms of IBS. Buy them when they're still hard and let them ripen at room temperature for a few days. Pure pear juice and dried pears are also helpful in treating this intestinal woe.

PEPPERMINT. Steeped into a nice, relaxing tea, this can relieve intestinal spasms. Use 1 heaping teaspoon dried peppermint, and steep in 1 cup boiling water for ten minutes. Drink as often as necessary.

YOGURT. Yogurt with active cultures will supply your digestive tract with the helpful kind of bacteria, which can ease IBS symptoms. You can also try mixing 1 cup yogurt with ½ teaspoon psyllium husks (or psyllium bulk you can buy in any pharmacy) and eating the mixture one hour after meals.

MORE DO'S & DON'TS

- Make sure you get enough fiber. It helps maintain good bowel function. You need about 35 grams a day. Chances are you're only getting about half of what you need.

- Limit alcohol and caffeine. They irritate your stomach lining, which can lead to IBS symptoms.

- Nix the tobacco. It can cause stomach cramps, among other deadly things.

- Skip the gassy foods. For a list of gassy foods, see page 96. And try to eliminate air swallowing. The more gas you introduce into your intestine, the more likely a flare-up of IBS.

- Drink between meals, not with meals. Drinking when you eat dilutes digestive juices and frustrates digestion.

- Avoid anything that causes stress. Relax during mealtimes. Give yourself plenty of time to complete your tasks. Avoid the morning rush-rush hassle by getting up a few minutes earlier. Spend a few minutes alone, working on progressive relaxation.

 # NO-NO FOODS

You may have your own personal list of foods that cause your IBS flare-ups, but these are a common cause, too:

- Dairy products
- Cereals, especially wheat cereals
- Red kidney beans
- Lentils

- Peas
- Apples
- Grapes
- Raisins
- Brussels sprouts

- Broccoli
- Cauliflower
- Preserved, processed, or cured meats

LACTOSE INTOLERANCE

Lactose, the milk sugar in dairy products, can be pretty rough to digest on a good day. But our bodies manage to do it with the help of an enzyme called lactase that breaks down those tough milk sugars and converts them into glucose, or blood sugar. When lactase kicks in, milk digestion comes off without a hitch.

When there is an insufficient amount of lactase, your condition is called lactose intolerance, and it can cause some pretty miserable symptoms. Instead of being broken down, lactose instead stays intact in the intestines, absorbing fluids. When this happens, gas, cramping, heartburn, and diarrhea can result one by one or all together. To add insult to injury, certain bacteria that call the colon home ferment the undigested lactose, causing more gas, cramping, and diarrhea.

A COMMON PROBLEM

Lactose intolerance is so common that about two-thirds of the world's population suffers from it in some form. This includes:

- About 50 million Americans
- 75 percent of African American, Jewish, Native American, and Mexican American adults
- 90 percent of Asian Americans

Globally, Native Americans, Africans, and people of Mediterranean, Asian, and Middle Eastern descent have the highest incidence of lactose intolerance. However, only 10 to 15 percent of non-Jewish Caucasian American adults suffer from it.

Most adults who are lactose intolerant usually tolerated small amounts of lactose when they were children. With aging, however, the ability to digest lactose diminishes, even for those who aren't lactose intolerant. To some degree, lactose intolerance develops in virtually everyone as they age. In other words, the body's production of lactase slows down, or ages, too.

Many people don't realize they're lactose intolerant, especially if they don't consume many milk products. Since the degree of intolerance varies with each individual, some may experience symptoms only after consuming a large amount of dairy. Others will have symptoms from a very small amount. One way to get some idea of whether you're lactose intolerant is simply to avoid all dairy products for several weeks and see if your symptoms resolve. This isn't a conclusive method, as there may be other reasons that your symptoms don't entirely disappear. But if your symptoms do decrease, you will benefit by decreasing dairy in your diet, using a dietary aid that replaces lactase (available in most pharmacies), or using a lactose-free milk product.

For a more conclusive diagnosis, visit your doctor, who may want to order a lactose intolerance test.

But before you get too discouraged, here are some easy remedies you can try to get some relief.

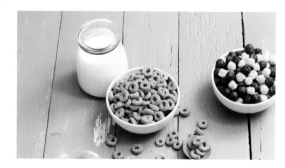

KITCHEN CURES

BUTTERMILK. It's more digestible than regular cow's milk. So is goat's milk.

COCOA POWDER. Studies indicate that cocoa powder and sugar, or chocolate powders, may help the body digest lactose by slowing the rate at which the stomach empties. The slower the emptying process, the less lactose that enters your system at once. That means fewer symptoms.

HARD CHEESE. Cheddar and Colby are good: The harder the cheese, the lower its lactose content. Skip the soft cheese, including cream cheese, cottage cheese, and any product that's processed or spreadable.

FOOD. People with any degree of lactose intolerance should never drink milk by itself. Always have a snack with your milk or have it with a meal.

SARDINES. They're high in calcium, which might be lacking in your diet if you're not drinking milk or consuming calcium-rich milk products. These foods are also high in calcium: canned salmon (or any other canned oily fish with bones), tofu, dark green leafy vegetables, nuts, cooked dried beans, dried apricots, and sesame seed products.

SOY MILK. It's a shock after you're used to cow's milk, but it won't cause lactose intolerance. If you can't get used to the taste, try using it in recipes and products such as pudding where adding milk is required.

YOGURT. Research shows that yogurt with active cultures may be a good source of calcium for many people with lactose intolerance, even though it is fairly high in lactose. According to the National Digestive Diseases Information Clearinghouse, evidence shows that the bacterial cultures used in making yogurt produce some of the lactase enzyme required for proper digestion.

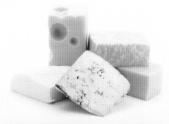

145

UNMASKING THE MILK

These all may contain milk that you're not aware of:

- Bread
- Cereals
- Pancakes
- Chocolate
- Pudding

- Soups, especially cream-based
- Salad dressing
- Sherbet
- Instant cocoa mix

- Soft candy
- Frozen dinners
- Cookie mix
- Hot dogs

The amounts may be negligible, but if you're very sensitive to lactose, even the tiny amounts of milk can cause symptoms.

TOOLS FROM THE DRAWER

MAGNIFYING GLASS. Check the product content listed on the label for hidden milk. The print may be tiny, but looking for milk could save you from misery. These are the buzzwords to look for: whey, curds, milk by-products, dry milk solids, nonfat dry milk, milk powder, milk sugar, casein, galactose, skim whey protein concentrate.

MEASURING CUP. Most people who suffer lactose intolerance do produce an amount of lactase. So, if that 8-ounce glass of milk you drink in the morning backfires, divide it up. Measure out $^1/_3$ cup three times a day and see if you can handle the smaller amount.

NOTEBOOK. Keep a food diary. First, cut out all milk products for 3 to 4 weeks. Then, add back small amounts of milk at a meal, $^1/_4$ to $^1/_2$ cup at a time, and see what you can tolerate. Gradually increase or decrease the amount according to your symptoms.

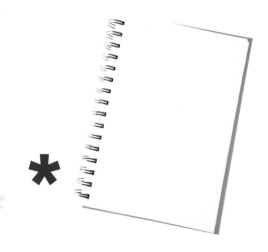

JUST PLAIN YOGURT

Originally produced as a way to preserve milk, yogurt is one of the most digestive tract-friendly foods you can eat, and its intestinal benefits have been recorded since the 16th century. The following yogurt facts pertain to regular yogurt with live cultures, not to yogurt products such as frozen treats.

- One cup a day can reduce total cholesterol by more than three percent.
- It fights the harmful bacteria responsible for diarrhea. Studies indicate that those who eat only yogurt during a severe bout may recover twice as quickly as those who are treated medically or by other means.
- It has a similar effect on the colon as fiber and can be used to maintain bowel regularity or relieve constipation.
- It's a good source of calcium and can be used in place of milk by those who are lactose intolerant because the bacteria in yogurt produce lactase.
- It helps relieve the symptoms of irritable bowel syndrome.
- A 1 $\frac{3}{4}$ cup serving has the same amount of calcium as about 4 cups milk.

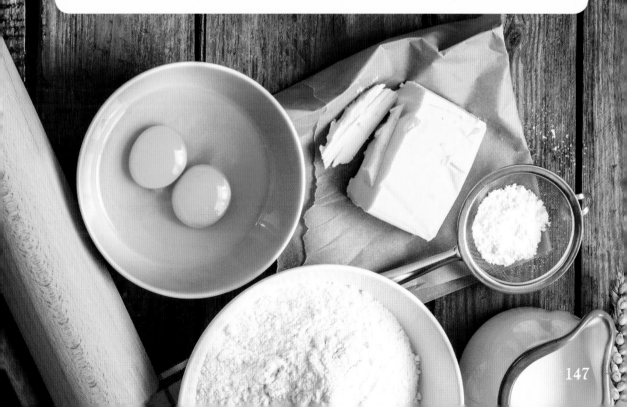

LOW IMMUNITY

In medical terms, having immunity means that you have resistance to infection or a specified disease. So if you have low immunity, it means your immune system isn't up to par and that you have a greater chance of getting the germ-du-jour. There are many factors that affect your body's response to a foreign invader, including how you're feeling at the moment you're introduced to a suspect germ. But if you consistently end up with the latest flu bug or stomach virus, your immune system may be running on empty.

THE BATTLE FOR YOUR BODY

Imagine your immune system as the front line in your body's war against foreign invaders. The vast network of glands, tissues, and cells are all soldiers working together to get rid of bacteria, viruses, parasites, and anything that invades their turf. The major troops in this war are the lymphatic system, made of the lymph nodes, thymus, spleen, and tonsils; white blood cells; and other specialized cells such as macrophages and mast cells. Each of these troops has a specialized job in enhancing the body's ability to fight off infection.

Lymph nodes are responsible for filtering out waste products from tissues throughout the body. Under the lymph nodes' command are cells that overtake bacteria and other potentially harmful foreign bodies and crush them like ants. That's why your lymph nodes swell up like golf balls when you are actively fighting off an infection.

The thymus is your immune system's stealth warfare command center. You may not have heard of the thymus, but without it you would be one sick puppy. The thymus is a gland that produces many of those disease-fighting foot soldiers—the white blood cells that come to your defense against many types of infections. And the thymus produces hormones that enhance your immune function overall. So if your thymus isn't working as it should, your body may have trouble fighting off infection.

The spleen is vital to your immune defense. It produces white blood cells, kills bacteria, and enhances the immune system overall. White blood cells are your body's main defense in the battle against infection. White blood cells with names such as neutrophils, eosinophils, basophils, T cells, B cells, and natural killer cells, are all part of the vast army of disease assaulters.

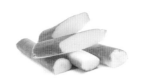 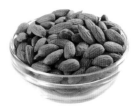

WHEN THE ENEMY STRIKES

When something enters your body that is viewed by the immune system as harmful, your body goes into a state of heightened alert. When your immune system is healthy and all systems are go, these foreign invaders, or antigens, are typically met by a barrage of antibodies, which are produced by white blood cells. These antibodies latch on to antigens and set into action all the events that lead to the invader's eventual demise.

If things in your immune system are not working properly, you become less able to fight off those foreign invaders. Eventually they set up shop in your body and you get sick. An impaired immune system can make you more susceptible to colds and other merely frustrating illnesses, but it can also make you more at risk for developing cancer.

Science is proving that getting enough of the right nutrients can help you build your immune system. Scientific studies are discovering that avoiding something as simple as a cold or something as life threatening as cancer may all be affected by what you stock in your kitchen.

KITCHEN CURES

ALMONDS. Eat a handful of almonds for your daily dose of vitamin E. An immune-strengthening antioxidant, studies have found that vitamin E deficiency causes major problems in the integrity of the immune system.

CARROTS. Carotenes, like the beta-carotene found in carrots and other red, yellow, orange, and dark-green leafy vegetables, are the protectors of the immune system, specifically the thymus gland. Carotenes strengthen white blood cell production, and numerous studies have shown that eating foods rich in beta-carotene helps the body fight off infection more easily.

CHICKEN. Selenium is a trace mineral that is vital to the development and movement of white blood cells in the body. A 3-ounce piece of chicken will give you almost half your daily needs.

CRAB. A zinc deficiency can zap your immune system. Zinc acts as a catalyst in the immune system's killer response to foreign bodies, and it protects the body from damage from invading cells. It also is a necessary ingredient for white blood cell function. Nosh on 3 ounces fresh or canned crab and you've got one-third of your recommended daily allowance (RDA) of this immune-enhancing nutrient.

GARLIC. Garlic is well-known for its antibacterial and antiviral properties. It's even been thought to help prevent cancer. Researchers think these benefits stem from garlic's amazing effect on the immune system. One study found that people who ate more garlic had more of the natural killer white blood cells than those who didn't eat garlic.

GUAVA. Go a little tropical with this tasty fruit and get more than twice your daily vitamin C needs. Vitamin C acts as an immune enhancer by helping white blood cells perform at their peak and quickening the response time of the immune system.

KALE. A cup of kale will give you your daily requirement of vitamin A. Vitamin A is an antioxidant that helps your body fight cancer cells and is essential in the formation of white blood cells. Vitamin A also increases the ability of antibodies to respond to invaders.

NAVY BEANS. Everybody needs a little folic acid (it's the most common nutrient deficiency in the United States). And not getting enough of this vital nutrient can actually shrink vital immune system fighters like your thymus and lymph nodes. To make sure you're getting your fill of folic acid, try popping open a can of navy beans with dinner. One cup gets you half of your recommended daily allowance (RDA) of folic acid.

PORK. Not getting enough vitamin B6 can keep your immune system from functioning at its best. Eating 3 ounces of lean roast pork will provide you with one-third of most adults' daily requirements for this immune-helping vitamin.

SHIITAKE MUSHROOMS. Throw a few shiitake mushrooms in your stir-fry and you may prevent your yearly cold. Scientists have discovered that specific components of shiitake mushrooms boost your immune system and act as antiviral agents.

YOGURT. Yogurt seems to have a marked effect on the immune system. It strengthens white blood cells and helps the immune system produce antibodies. One study found that people who ate 6 ounces of yogurt a day avoided colds, hay fever, and diarrhea. Another study found that yogurt could be a ally in the body's war against cancer.

 # FOODS TO AVOID

- Skip the sugar. Sugar may keep your white blood cells from being their strongest. Keep the sweet stuff to a minimum if your immune system isn't working like it should.

- Forgo fat. Polyunsaturated fats in vegetable oils such as corn, safflower, and sunflower oil seem to be a deterrent to an efficiently running immune system.

MENOPAUSE

Well, "Aunt Flo" won't be making her monthly visit any more. The baby factory is closed. You won't be indisposed or down with the "flu" or under the weather for those few days every month. Most women look forward to the cessation of menstruation and all its associated annoyances. It happens to every woman sometime between the ages of 40 and 60, and on average at age 51. But menopause isn't just closing the door on Aunt Flo. It's a process of bodily changes and a reduction in female hormones, and it occurs over several years.

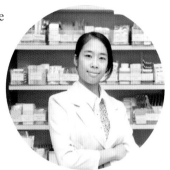

These are some of the pre-menopausal changes:

- Estrogen levels begin to drop off around age 30.

- Egg production and release slow down, usually during the 40s.

- Menstrual cycles change. They become longer or shorter, lighter or heavier. Months— or only a week or two—may elapse between periods.

- Whatever happens this time will change next time.

Overall, it takes about four years to get through these changes and cross that menopause threshold, but once menstruation has been absent for a full year, you are pronounced "postmenopausal."

In the meantime, as menopause is galloping to the finishing line, it's dragging along a lot of symptoms: hot flashes, vaginal dryness, bladder infection, incontinence, heart palpitations, achy joints, dry or itchy skin, headache, insomnia, weight gain, thinning hair, increased facial hair, mood swings, memory problems, and change in sexual drive.

Obviously, this transition requires some medical guidance, since the consequences can be much more serious than the profuse sweating of a hot flash. But there are ways to curb some of the menopausal symptoms right in your own kitchen. And since menopause is nothing to cure, but rather to endure, curbing those problems so simply can be a big relief.

KITCHEN CURES

ALFALFA SPROUTS. Their plant estrogen may help prevent thinning of the vaginal walls. Sprinkle on a salad or use in a stir-fry. Make sure your sprouts are clean before you eat them, though. Raw sprouts can be contaminated with the *E. coli* bacteria. Flaxseed is rich in natural estrogen, too.

LIME JUICE. Mix 5 to 10 drops with 1 teaspoon organic sugar and 1 cup pomegranate juice. Drink two to three times a day to relieve hot flashes.

ORANGES. The vitamin C in oranges is a natural immune booster. It also guards your skin against damage. Other C-rich foods include grapefruits, berries, papayas, green leafy veggies, peppers, and sweet potatoes.

PARSLEY. Joint aches and pains are a common complaint of menopause and parsley tea may bring relief. Steep a spoonful in a cup of boiling water for ten minutes, sweeten to taste, and drink two to three times a day. If you can stand the strong taste, add more parsley.

SAGE. This has estrogenlike properties and can help reduce sweating and hot flashes. Steep 1 to 2 fresh leaves or a spoonful of dried sage in 1 cup boiling water for ten minutes. Sweeten with honey, add lemon if desired. Drink a cup or two every day. Or, use sage as a spice on vegetables or to season meats.

SARDINES. Canned sardines, with bones and oil, are rich in bone-building calcium. Because loss of bone density is a common companion to menopause and can lead to osteoporosis, calcium-rich foods are important. Low fat dairy foods, sesame seeds, nuts, and legumes also should be added to your diet.

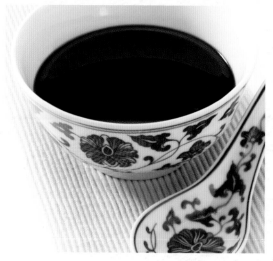

SOY. It comes in many forms and they're all great at relieving symptoms such as hot flashes and vaginal dryness, preventing loss of bone density, and lowering cholesterol. Try adding tofu, soy milk, and tempeh to your diet.

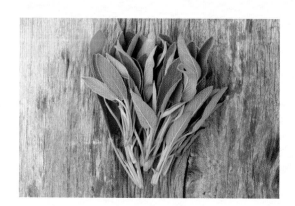

MEMORY PROBLEMS

Some events, and some names and faces, definitely should be forgotten. Embarrassing moments, things you wish you hadn't said or done, are memories you can relegate to the memory trash bin. Purposely forgetting is one thing, and we all try to do it on occasion. But on those occasions when memory simply fails you—when you truly don't remember a name, a job assignment slips your mind, you forget a doctor's appointment—your forgetfulness can have unpleasant consequences.

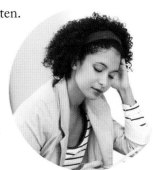

Forgetting is normal. We all experience it from time to time. And when it's an occasional problem, that's OK. But when forgetfulness becomes a chronic problem, that indicates that one of two things is happening:

1. You're not locking in the information you just received. New information will be lost in seven seconds if you don't lock it in right away.

2. You have a physical or mental condition that's preventing you from remembering. For example: Alzheimer's disease, senile dementia, hypoglycemia, severe anemia, depression, anxiety, alcohol or drug abuse, head injury, or severe viral or bacterial illness. Some prescribed medications make remembering a little difficult, too.

Memory is divided into two parts: short-term and long-term. The short-term memory bank holds the memory for only a few seconds, then transfers it to the long-term memory bank. If the transfer doesn't take place, the memory is lost.

If you're affected by the Seven-Second Syndrome, which is failing to lock in information once it's presented to you, there are memory-strengthening techniques that can improve that forgetfulness.

Sometimes memory problems stem from nutritional deficiencies, stress, and other problems that can be controlled once you know how. Here are some KMBs—kitchen memory boosters—that might just help you remember.

KITCHEN CURES

ANISEED. Some herbalists suggest using aniseed to improve memory. Add 7 teaspoons aniseed to 1 quart boiling water, and let it simmer until it reduces by about half. Strain, and while still warm, add 4 teaspoons honey and 4 teaspoons glycerine, which can be purchased at the drugstore. Take 2 tablespoons three times.

ARTICHOKES. These are thought to increase your mental acuity. Prepare and eat them as you normally would or follow this recipe for an elixir of artichoke: Pull the artichoke apart, leaf by leaf, then put the pieces into a jar and add enough water to just barely cover. Cover the jar with a lid or saucer, and place in a pan with water. Boil for two hours, adding more water to the pan (not the jar) as necessary. Then strain the contents of the jar and give the artichoke leaves a good squeeze to get out all the juices. Take 3 to 4 tablespoons four times a day.

BLUEBERRIES. These luscious little fruits are the richest source of antioxidants, and recent studies have shown that blueberries may help improve short-term memory. Strawberries and cherries are good, too.

CARROTS. They contain carotene, which is a memory booster. Eat them raw, cooked, or in casseroles, or make a juice with carrots and apricots. The apricots are used to add a little compatible juice to the dry carrots.

EGGS. These have lecithin, which keeps the memory nerve cells healthy. Lecithin is also found in sunflower and soybean oils and can be purchased in capsule form, too. Studies indicate that taking up to 70 grams a day may improve memory.

OKRA. If not a memorable food, this is at least a memory-enhancing food. So are sweet potatoes, tapioca, and spinach. Fresh fruits, especially oranges, and vegetables, almonds, and milk are also good for stimulating the memory.

PISTACHIO NUTS. If your memory loss is the result of a thiamine deficiency, pistachio nuts can help. One of the richest sources of thiamine, $1/2$ cup supplies 0.54 mg of thiamin. The RDA for thiamine is 1.5 mg for men and 1.1 for women age 50 and younger; slightly less for those over 50.

WHEAT GERM. Wheat germ is a good source of vitamin E, which may help with age-related memory loss.

FROM THE SUPPLEMENT SHELF

VITAMIN B6. A deficiency in this vitamin, also called pyridoxine, can cause memory loss. Supplementation may improve memory in older adults.

VITAMIN E. Recent studies have reported improved short-term memory in older adults who took supplemental vitamin E.

MENSTRUAL PROBLEMS

Ah, that time of the month again. It seems as if it rolls around about every other day, doesn't it? When you were young, anticipating your very first period, you were excited by that passage into woman- hood. But you didn't anticipate the inconvenience, pain, and all the associated problems: bloat, backache, leg aches, headaches, zits, cramps, and mood swings. And those are on a good menstrual day. On a bad day, bleeding is so heavy you can't move without gushing or you're too tired to breathe. When you figure out that it's more of an inconvenience than something to look forward to, you've joined the true menses sisterhood.

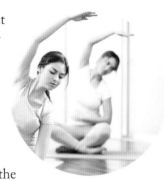

Menstruation is the simple process of shedding the old uterine lining to make way for a new one. In other words, it's the body's way of sweeping out the cobwebs at the end of the month in preparation for the arrival of a new egg and a new cycle; all a part of the natural baby-mak- ing process with one goal in mind: conception.

Who experiences menstrual problems? At one time or another, every woman who menstru- ates. But some factors make problems more likely. **These include:**

- Family history of problems
- Being overweight
- Being severely underweight, also linked with amenorrhea, as is being an athlete
- Taking certain drugs
- Chemotherapy or radiation

Most women will experience in the neighborhood of 400 menstrual cycles in their childbear- ing lifetime. And that's a lot of cycles that can cause problems. Serious menstrual problems require medical treatment, since many can lead to infertility, infection, and in some cases, death. But some of the milder problems can be relieved with simple kitchen cures. And any menstrual relief, no matter how slight, is welcome!

KITCHEN CURES

BASIL. This can relieve some of the normal pain associated with menstruation because it contains caffeic acid, which has an analgesic, or pain-killing, effect. Thyme is also high in caffeic acid. Use it as a spice in cooking meat and vegetables or Italian dishes. Or steep the herb into tea, adding 2 tablespoons thyme or basil leaves to 1 pint boiling water. Cover tightly and let cool to room temperature. Drink $^1\!/_2$ to 1 cup an hour for painful menstruation.

BUCKWHEAT. It's high in bioflavonoids and can reduce heavy bleeding when taken with vitamin C. Try it in buckwheat pancakes. Fruits, nuts, and seeds are high in bioflavonoids, too.

CINNAMON. This has anti-inflammatory and antispasmodic properties that relieve cramps. Use as a tea, or sprinkle on toast or sweet rolls. If you have a heavy period, drinking cinnamon tea the day before or during your period may help.

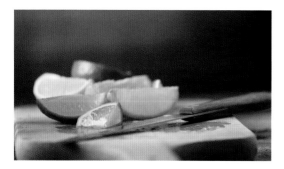

CITRUS FRUITS. Eat or drink with your meals to enhance iron absorption into the body, since iron is easily depleted during menstruation.

DRIED APRICOTS. These are high in iron, which is important during menstruation because iron supplies can be depleted with heavy bleeding. Other iron-rich foods are: liver, legumes, shellfish, and fortified breads and cereals.

FENNEL. Another cramp cure, this spice promotes better circulation to the ovaries. Crush 1 teaspoon fennel seeds into a powder. Add to 1 cup boiling water, steep five minutes, strain, and drink hot.

GINGER. This is a cramp reliever, and as an added bonus it sometimes can make irregular periods regular. Use in cookies, cake, and candy or as a spice in vegetables and stir-fries. Tea may be the most effective form, however: put $^1\!/_2$ teaspoon in 1 cup boiling water, and drink three times a day.

HOT WATER. Put it in a hot water bottle and place on the abdomen to relieve cramps. Or, soak a kitchen towel, then wring out excess water, heat in microwave for a minute, and place on abdomen. Be careful not to burn yourself.

MINT. Either peppermint or wintergreen can relieve cramps. Steep into a tea and drink a cup or two a day. Try sucking on mint candy, too.

MUSTARD. A tablespoon or two of powdered mustard in a basin of nice warm water can relieve cramps, but don't drink it. Soak your feet in it to reap the relaxing effects.

RED MEAT. It's loaded with iron as well as zinc, which can be depleted during menses, too. Zinc is necessary for healthy bones, and a zinc deficiency may result in amenorrhea. Other iron- and zinc-rich foods: poultry, fish, green leafy vegetables.

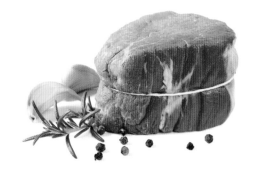

WATER. Drink plenty of it. Dehydration can cause the body to produce a hormone called vasopressin that contributes to cramps.

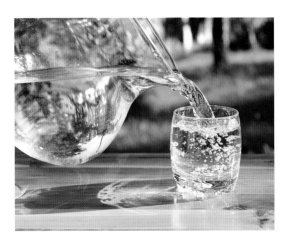

FROM THE SUPPLEMENT SHELF

Women who have heavy periods may find relief by taking vitamin K supplements. This is the case even if the blood levels of the vitamin are within the normal range.

HERBAL CURES

Typically, the cure for female complaints has been one or more herbs. Some of the more common are found in most spice racks, but here are a few you might wish to seek out to stock that menstrual medicinal herb rack.

Chamomile. This is known to be a reliable cramp reliever. Place $1/2$ ounce in a 1-pint jar and cover with boiling water. Steep for one hour, strain, and drink a cup every hour or two. Use honey to sweeten to taste. This is a particularly relaxing tea just before bed.

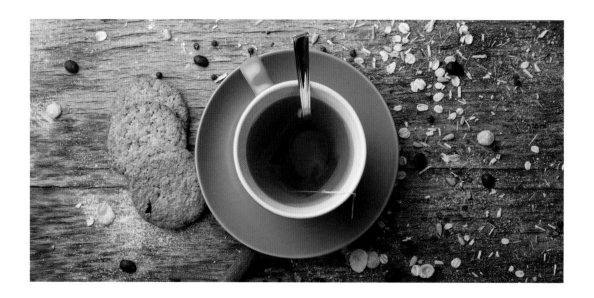

Juniper Berries. Steeped into a tea, this can bring on delayed menstruation. Crush 1 teaspoon juniper berries in a coffee grinder or food processor. Place 1 teaspoon of the powder into a cup and fill with boiling water. Steep ten minutes, then take $1/4$ cup doses every three to four hours. Do not take this tea if you have kidney disease, or for more than three weeks. **Warning! Juniper berries can cause spontaneous abortion.**

Lemon balm. This is another cramp reliever, also used for menstruation delayed by stress and tension. Lemon balm also has a mild sedative effect. Make the tea by placing 1 ounce of the herb in 1 quart boiling water, then letting it cool to room temperature. Strain and drink $1/2$ cup per hour until the cramps are gone.

Motherwort. This herb has a folk use in curing menstrual cramps and delayed menstruation, and it has sedative proper-

ties that can relieve stress or nervousness. Place $1/2$ ounce of the dried flowering tops in a 1-pint jar and cover with boiling water. Let stand for 20 minutes, then strain and rebottle. Take 1 to 2 ounces of the tea every two to three hours for up to three days. Do not use if you are taking a medication for a thyroid or heart condition. Do not use if menstrual bleeding is heavy.

Raspberry leaf. Place 1 ounce raspberry leaf in 1 pint water, then bring to a slow boil. Cover and simmer on the lowest heat 30 to 40 minutes. Cool, stir, strain, bottle. Sweeten to taste. One raspberry leaf contains: 408 mg calcium, 446 mg potassium, 106 mg magnesium, 4 mg manganese, and 3.3 mg iron.

Yarrow. A tea made with this herb can stop excessive or prolonged bleeding. It can be taken during the period for bleeding relief or at the beginning to make the entire period easier.

MOTION SICKNESS

It can happen almost anywhere—in the backseat of your family van, on the Tilt-a-Whirl at the county fair, on the bumpy airplane ride to grandma's. Anything that moves has the potential to give you a green hue and leave you wishing the world would put on the brakes. Anyone who has experienced motion sickness would agree that it is a horrible feeling—one they wouldn't want to make a repeat appearance. Thankfully, most people only deal with motion sickness on occasion. And following some simple tips can help avert those rare bouts.

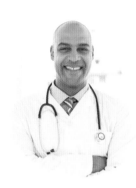

TUMMY TURBULENCE

So why does your tummy do cartwheels every time you sail, fly, or ride? Motion sickness is purely a matter of miscommunication. When you're cruising down the road focused on a book or a person, your eyes tell your brain that you're not moving, but your inner ear tells the brain a different story. For instance, you and your girlfriends are going for a long-awaited women-only weekend. All six of you pile in your friend's minivan. You pop in the passenger seat and as soon as you get on the road, you're turned around chatting with your buddies. You see only your stationary friends sitting in the back of the van, so your eyes tell your brain that you're sitting in a room catching up with old pals. But the fluid in your inner ear is sloshing around with every bump and turn. Your brain is getting mixed signals. And in the confusion, your brain triggers your tummy and you start feeling sick. Next thing you know, you and the girls are forced to make a pit stop.

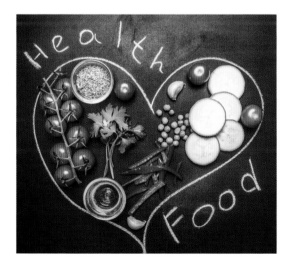

SYMPTOMS OF A SPINNING HEAD

No one can completely avoid motion sickness. Even astronauts have bouts of nausea every now and then. For most people, motion sickness comes on fairly quickly and usually involves one of these symptoms: sweating, hyperventilation, dizziness, paleness, sensation of spinning, loss of appetite, and of course, nausea.

KITCHEN CURES

APPLE JUICE. Drink a glass of apple juice with your pre-travel low fat meal. Giving your body a bit of sugar with fluids before you start your journey should help you down the road. And if you start feeling ill, sipping (not gulping) some juice may help you feel better. Almost any non-citrus juice will do. Citrus juice irritates an already un-stable stomach.

CRACKERS. Take these easily digestible snacks along and nibble on them every couple of hours to help prevent nausea and vomiting. An empty stomach makes it more likely that you will get sick.

GINGER. Ginger has long been known as an herbal remedy for queasiness, but mod-ern science has proved this spice has merit, especially for motion sickness. One study discovered that ginger was actually better than over-the-counter motion sickness drugs. Make a ginger tea to take along with you when you're traveling by cutting 10 to 12 slices of fresh ginger and placing them in a pot with 1 quart water. Boil for ten minutes. Strain out the ginger, and add ½ cup honey or maple syrup for sweetening if you like.

LOW FAT FOODS. If you eat a low fat meal before you head out on your trip, you may avoid getting sick. Eating something before you leave makes your stomach more capable of handling the ups and downs of the road. Experts say not eating destabilizes the

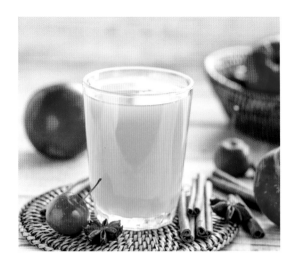

stomach's electrical signals, making you sus-ceptible to nausea and vomiting.

PEPPERMINT CANDIES OR LOZENGES. If you start feeling sick, get out the pepper-mints. Not only will you end up with fresh minty breath when you arrive at your desti-nation, you'll also calm your queasiness. And if you're traveling with little ones, try plac-ing 1 drop peppermint oil on their tongues before the trip. It may quash the queasies.

TEA. Sip on some warm tea if you start feeling sick. Warm beverages tend to be easier on a nauseated tummy than a tall glass of cold water. Go for the decaf brew; caffeinated drinks aren't a good idea for un-stable stomachs.

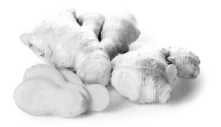

MUSCLE SORENESS AND CRAMPING

You've made your New Year's resolution: You are going to get in shape. Never mind that the last time you exercised was at a charity walk a few years ago and that the very expensive treadmill you bought is now buried underneath a pile of laundry. Twenty pounds and three kids ago you were an aerobics queen, so you know what it's like to feel, and look, better. So you venture into your local health club and decide to try the low/high aerobics class for people who have been out of circulation for a while. You think you can keep up with the twenty-something girls, so you grapevine and kick and half-jack with the beat for 50 minutes. By the time you get home, though, your muscles have gone on strike. The next day you can barely muster enough strength to make it out of bed, and you spend the day walking like you've been riding the range a bit too long. You'll take it slower next time. But what can you do right now to ease the pain?

MUSCLE MAYHEM

The vast array of muscles in your body is what allows you to do something as simple as picking up a fork or as complicated as a kickboxing routine. Muscles are a complex weave of fibers that work with your brain and skeletal system to give you the agility to return that volley across the tennis court. When you're taking care to stretch and strengthen your muscles, they are your greatest ally. But when they don't work like they should or they get injured, you have a very painful problem on your hands.

Strains are one of the most common reasons for aching muscles. When you strain a muscle, it means you've worked it too hard, causing the muscle fibers to pull and tear. If you haven't worked out for a while and then head back full throttle without preparing your muscles for the trauma they're about to experience, or if you're an experienced exerciser and you don't warm up properly, you risk getting a strained muscle. At best, a strained muscle will leave you sore for a few days; at worst, you could end up with a "pulled" muscle, one whose fibers have been totally torn.

Another common muscle malady is cramps, or spasms. Muscle cramps happen when the muscle isn't getting enough blood, and in response to the restricted blood flow the muscle shortens and tightens. The slowdown in blood flow can be caused by a variety of problems:

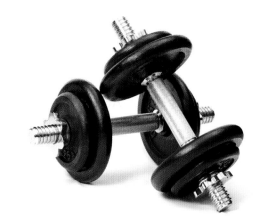

- A deficiency in essential nutrients for maximum muscle power, such as sodium, calcium, and potassium

- Depletion of the muscles' energy supply of glycogen

- Overworked muscles

- Holding the same position for too long

KITCHEN CURES

BANANA. Eat a banana or two a day and you may cut down your cramping. That's because a potassium deficiency may be to blame for muscle cramps. One banana has 450 mg of the muscle-protecting nutrient.

BOUILLON. Sipping some warm soup before heading out for a long bike ride may not sound appealing, but it may help you skip the muscle cramps. Drink 1 cup beef or chicken bouillon before you ride. It helps you replace the sodium you lose when you sweat.

MILK. Getting adequate amounts of calcium in your diet may help curtail your cramps. Women especially seem to need plenty of calcium for muscle health. Three glasses of milk a day will meet the calcium needs of most adults.

ROSEMARY. A few leaves of rosemary can help reduce swelling in strained muscles. Use either fresh or dried leaves; fresh has more of the volatile oils. The herb has four anti-inflammatory properties, which can help calm inflamed muscle tissue and speed healing. Because rosemary is easily absorbed through the skin, placing a cloth soaked with a rosemary wash will help ease the pain. Here's how to make a rosemary wash: Put 1 ounce rosemary leaves in a 1-pint jar and fill the jar with boiling water. Cover and let stand for 30 minutes. Apply the wash to the area two or three times a day.

SKIP THE SPORTS DRINKS.

Unless you're running more than an hour every day, you really don't need a sports drink. Water is your best bet for replacing fluids.

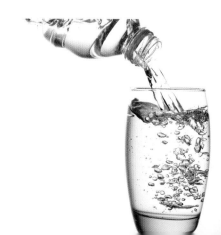

OSTEOPOROSIS

More than 28 million Americans are at risk for osteoporosis, and more than 10 million already have been diagnosed with this bone-degenerating disease. Women make up an astounding 80 percent of those who are affected by osteoporosis. Though most people associate osteoporosis with older people, the disease strikes young and old alike. But osteoporosis does become much more common as you age—affecting one in two women over age 50.

BONE UP ON OSTEOPOROSIS

As you grow your bones get stronger and longer. By the time you reach the age of 20, you've got 98 percent of your bone mass; by the time you reach your thirtieth birthday, your bones are their strongest. If you were able to take a look inside your bones during those peak years, you'd see a hard outer shell and something that looks like a honeycomb on the inside. About 80 percent of your bone mass is that tough, hard outer bone called cortical bone. The rest of your bone make-up is the honeycomblike material called trabecular bone. After you hit 30, your bone mass begins to decline. Trabecular bone is typically the first to lose critical density, and as you get older, cortical bone mass also declines, but at a slower pace.

Osteoporosis literally means porous bones. That means someone diagnosed with the disease has lost so much density that there's not much there to hold their bones together, putting them at greater risk for bone breaks and fractures. The National Osteoporosis Foundation calls osteoporosis the "silent disease" because there are virtually no symptoms of bone loss. Unless you're aware of the risk factors and take action, you may not know you have the disease until some benign bump on the garage door turns into a fracture.

WHO GETS OSTEOPOROSIS?

When you think of osteoporosis, you probably picture a petite, silver-haired Caucasian woman. And, in reality, that woman could be the poster child for the disease—being Caucasian or Asian, female, small-framed, and under-weight are major risk factors for thinning bones. And so is being postmenopausal. That's because estrogen is vital to bone strength, keeping bones strong by stimulating bone-building substances called osteoblasts and suppressing bone-destroying substances called osteoclasts. Estrogen also

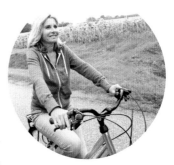

helps the body absorb and use calcium more efficiently. As women approach menopause, estrogen production steadily declines and the protection it provides against osteoporosis is lost. But one of the greatest risk factors for osteoporosis is something you can't see and you can't control—heredity. Other risk factors include: not getting enough calcium, having an eating disorder, using certain medications such as corticosteriods, not exercising, and smoking.

Thankfully, there are many ways you can combat and even reverse the damaging effects of this bone-thinning disease, and the earlier you start the better. Why not try some of the bone boosters in your kitchen?

KITCHEN CURES

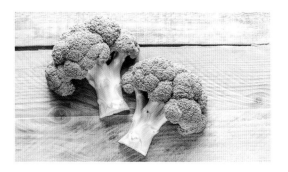

APPLES. Boron is a trace mineral that helps your body hold on to calcium—the building block of bones. It even acts as a mild estrogen replacement, and losing estrogen is instrumental in speeding bone loss. Boron is found in apples and other fruits such as pears, grapes, dates, raisins, and peaches. It's also in nuts such as almonds, peanuts, and hazelnuts.

BANANA. Eat a banana a day to build your bones. Studies have found that women who have diets high in potassium also have stronger bones in their spines and hips. Researchers think this is related to potassium's ability to keep blood healthy and balanced so the body doesn't have to suck calcium from the skeleton to keep blood up to par.

BROCCOLI. Eat $^1/_2$ cup broccoli to get your daily dose of vitamin K. Studies are finding that postmenopausal women with low levels of this vital vitamin are more likely to have osteoporosis.

MARGARINE. Slather a teaspoon of low trans fatty margarine on your toast for a dose of vitamin D. Vitamin D helps the body absorb calcium, a necessary ingredient to bone health.

MILK. When it comes to strong bones, getting enough calcium is a must. One cup of milk can provide 300 mg of the 1,000 to 1,200 mg of calcium the government recommends you get every day. But milk is not the only calcium-rich food on the market. See "Mooove Over Milk," on page 166, for more ideas on how to add this bone-strengthening mineral to your diet.

ORANGE JUICE. Grab a glass of OJ to get your vitamin C. Necessary for the body processes that rebuild bones, getting enough vitamin C is vital to preventing osteoporosis. Grab some calcium-fortified orange juice and get a healthy dose of bone-building nutrients.

PEANUT BUTTER. A recent review of studies on nutrition and osteoporosis found that magnesium was a vital component to strengthening, preserving, and rebuilding bones. You can get 50 mg of magnesium by eating 2 tablespoons of peanut butter.

PINEAPPLE JUICE. Drink a cup of pineapple juice and give your body some manganese. Studies are finding that manganese deficiency is a predictor of osteoporosis. Other manganese sources are oatmeal, nuts, beans, cereals, spinach, and tea.

TOFU. Soy is showing promise as a potential bone strengthener. Soy contains proteins that act like a weak estrogen in the body. These "phytoestrogens," or plant-based estrogens, may help women regain bone strength.

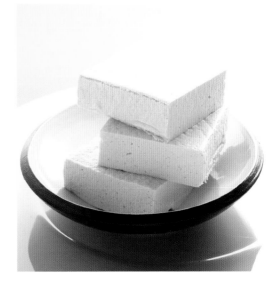

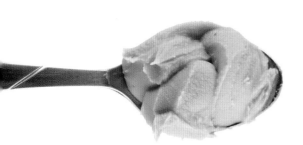

MORE DO'S AND DON'TS

- If you don't get enough calcium in your diet, be sure to use a supplement to help prevent osteoporosis.

- Restrict your salt. Salt may actually steal calcium away from your bones.

- Abstain from alcohol. Alcohol interferes with the way your body absorbs calcium.

- Cut the caffeine. Caffeine is a diuretic, and some experts believe drinking too much can cause your body to excrete too much calcium. Don't drink more than 2 cups of coffee or 4 cups of tea a day.

- Get some sun. To up your supply of vitamin D, be sure to catch a few rays. Spending 15 minutes a day in the sun will give you an adequate supply without causing your skin to suffer.

MOOOVE
OVER MILK

Milk isn't the only way you can load up on calcium. There are plenty of nondairy, calcium-rich foods out there. If you're lactose intolerant or simply don't like the taste of milk but you want to be sure you're getting enough calcium, check out these calcium-rich choices.

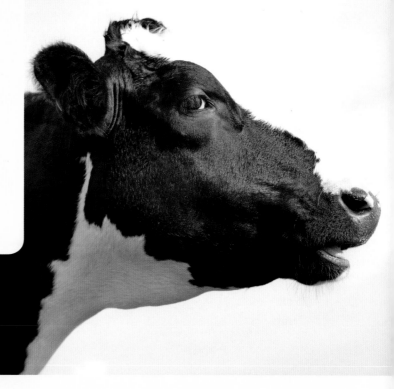

FOOD	CALCIUM CONTENT (MILLIGRAMS)
salmon, with bones (3 ounces)	205
blackstrap molasses (1 tablespoon)	185
tofu ($^1/_2$ cup)	130
turnip greens ($^1/_2$ cup)	100
dried figs (3)	80
okra ($^1/_2$ cup)	50
orange (1)	45

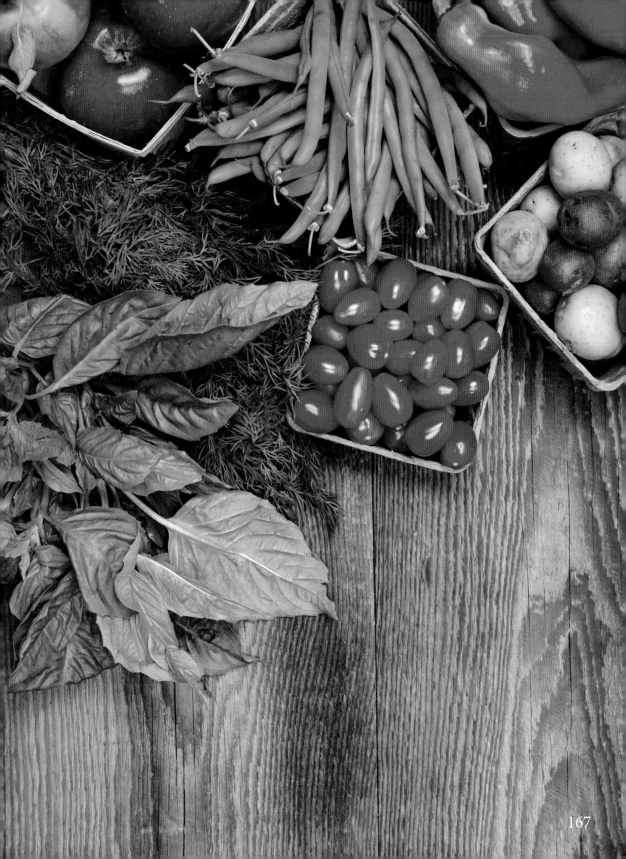

POOR APPETITE

What do you mean you're not hungry? You've probably heard this response when you declare no desire to eat. While the response may sound like nagging, it is an understandable one. Humans have a physical need for food and nourishment, so when an appetite is lacking, something is amiss...and that alarms people who care about you.

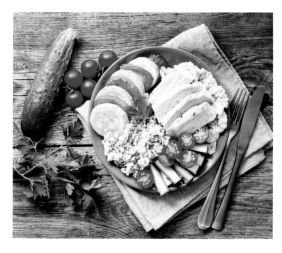

A poor appetite can stem from many factors. Perhaps the most common causes are emotional upset, nervousness, tension, anxiety, or depression. Stressful events, such as losing a job or a death in the family, can also make the appetite plummet. Diseases such as influenza and acute infections play a role in appetite reduction, as do anorexia nervosa and fatigue. Illegal and legal drugs, including amphetamines, antibiotics, cough and cold medications, codeine, morphine, and Demerol can take a toll on the appetite. Sometimes poor eating habits, such as continuous snacking, can lead to a poor appetite at mealtimes. A poor appetite can also be one symptom of a serious disease.

Fortunately, for minor cases of poor appetite, the kitchen is the best place to get the appetite back into gear.

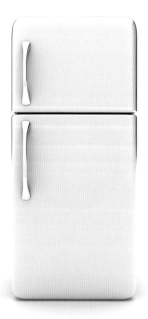

THE FRENCH CONNECTION

The culinary-minded French have a highly seasoned stew of meat or fish called ragout. The name is derived from the meaning, "to restore the appetite of."

KITCHEN CURES

BITTER GREENS. Mama always told you to eat your greens. If she knew you weren't eating properly, she might add, eat your "bitter" greens. Bitter greens consist of arugula, radicchio, collards, kale, endives, escarole, mizuna, sorrel, dandelions, watercress, and red/green mustard...in other words, all those leaves you find in fancy restaurant salads. Stimulating digestion is the name of the game with bitter greens. They prompt the body into making more digestive juices and digestive enzymes. Bitter foods also stimulate the gallbladder to contract and release bile, which helps break fatty foods into small enough particles that enzymes can easily finish breaking them apart for absorption. This is important because fats carry essential fatty acids, such as heart-healthy omega-3s, along with fat-soluble vitamins A, D, E, and K and carotenoids such as beta-carotene.

CARAWAY. The early Greeks knew caraway could calm an upset stomach and used it to season foods that were hard to digest. Today unsuspecting cooks who simply love the flavor of caraway continue the tradition by adding caraway to rye bread, cabbage dishes, sauerkraut and coleslaw, pork, cheese sauces, cream soups, goose, and duck. The Germans make a caraway liqueur called Kümmel and serve it after heavy meals. One of the easiest ways to enjoy caraway is with a good helping of sauerkraut. Sauté ¹/₂ medium onion in 1 to 2 tablespoons butter. When onions turn deep golden brown, add 1 can sauerkraut and its liquid along with 1 or 2 tablespoons brown sugar and 1 teaspoon caraway seeds. Let the mixture simmer (covered) for 1 hour. Serve as a side dish with meat, poultry, or sausage.

CAYENNE PEPPER. Nothing revs up the old digestive engine like cayenne. Cayenne pepper has the power to make any dish fiery hot, but it also has a subtle flavor-enhancing quality. There is some evidence that eating hot pepper increases metabolism and the appetite. Add a few shakes of cayenne pepper to potato salad, deviled eggs, chili, and other hot dishes such as stews and soups.

FENNEL. Fennel, like its cousin caraway (both belong to the Umbelliferae family of herbs), is a familiar digestive aid, both for relieving stomach upset and for boosting the appetite.

GINGER. Ginger helps stimulate a tired appetite, both through its medicinal properties and its refreshing taste. Try nibbling on gingersnaps or sipping ginger ale made with real ginger. Ginger tea is also a way to start the day off on an appetizing note. To make, place ¹/₂ teaspoon powdered ginger into a cup and fill with boiling water. Cover and let stand ten minutes. Strain and sip. Don't take more than three times daily. If needed, sweeten with just a little honey.

Warning! Pregnant women should consult a doctor before taking ginger.

MINT. Peppermint refreshes the palate and revives the appetite. Make a cup of mint tea and enjoy anytime you don't feel like eating. Place 1 tablespoon mint leaves in a 1-pint jar of boiling water. Let stand 20 to 30 minutes, shaking occasionally. Strain and sip as needed. If you're tired of teas, make a glass of mint lemonade by adding a few sprigs to the lemonade mixture and letting it sit for ten minutes before sipping.

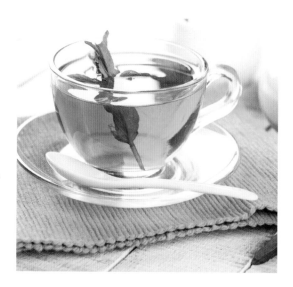

LOOK TO THE LAWN FOR HELP

Dandelions help stimulate digestion, thanks to a bitter substance called taraxacin that promotes the flow of bile from the liver and hydrochloric acid secretions from the stomach. Dandelion also helps the body to absorb nutrients and eliminate wastes more efficiently. Don't use dandelions from any lawns that may have been sprayed with chemicals or fertilizers. Dandelions are also available in some groceries and fruit and vegetable markets. Here is a recipe to get you started:

SAUTÉED DANDELIONS

Add young dandelions to your favorite stir-fry. Or sauté them with mushrooms, onions, and shredded kale and cabbage in some sesame oil. The greens cook quickly, even on low heat, so take care not to overcook. (They'll be mushy and distasteful if you do.) Remove from heat, add a dash of sesame oil and balsamic vinegar, and garnish with sesame seeds. Serve as a side dish or over rice.

Warning! Avoid dandelions if you have too much stomach acid, ulcers, diarrhea, irritable bowel syndrome, or ulcerative colitis.

HEAD HOME TO COMFORT FOODS

Sometimes a poor appetite can be remedied by those foods you adored during childhood: macaroni and cheese, mashed potatoes, green bean casserole, roast chicken, or a big slice of chocolate cake. A favorite dish or dessert can be just the cure you need to get yourself out of a digestive slump. Splurge on foods that make you feel better.

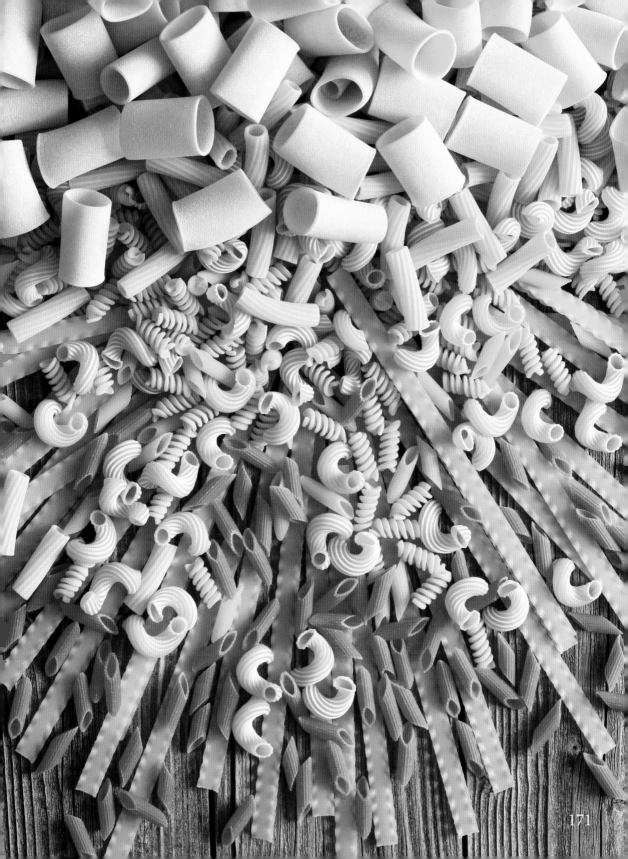

PREMENSTRUAL SYNDROME

That soon-to-be-time of the month, and all of a sudden you do the Jekyll-Hyde switch. Your mild, calm demeanor is replaced by rages, and your emotions become unstable. Sometimes you just feel out of control. At this time of the month, friends and loved ones may do their best to avoid you.

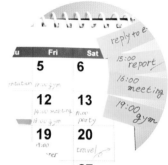

These mood swings, along with a host of other symptoms such as water retention, breast swelling and tenderness, depression, irritability, fatigue, food cravings, and headaches, are known as premenstrual syndrome (PMS). They typically begin a few days to a week before menstruation and end when the menstrual period begins.

Researchers believe that about 40 percent of women of child-bearing age experience PMS in some form. Symptoms and severity vary from mild and manageable to severe and disruptive. Some women only have one symptom, while others have a whole constellation of symptoms. But PMS can be downright brutal for about 15 percent of women. They're the ones who experience many symptoms to a debilitating degree, causing serious problems on the job and in interpersonal relationships.

WHAT CAUSES PMS?

Well, doctors don't really know what causes PMS, but they believe it is a result of hormonal changes, particularly in estrogen, that occur around the menstrual cycle. Some believe that PMS mood swings may be related to deficiencies in vitamin B6 and magnesium. One theory of PMS suggests that its symptoms are due to an ovarian hormone imbalance of either estrogen or progesterone.

Even though it's not fully understood, PMS is now recognized as a legitimate condition, not something that's all in women's heads. There are medications available that can mitigate or stop many of the harshest symptoms. Like so many other conditions, though, there are simple kitchen treatments that will work in relieving symptoms. So try them and see what happens. If you're a PMS sufferer, you know that anything that might help is worth a try.

KITCHEN CURES

AVOCADOS. These contain natural serotonin, which may supplement the mood-lifting brain chemical naturally produced by the body. Dates, plums, eggplants, papayas, plantains, and pineapple are also sources of serotonin.

BANANAS. Rich in potassium, they can relieve the bloating and swelling of water retention that comes with PMS. Other foods such as figs, black currants, potatoes, broccoli, onions, and tomatoes are potassium-rich, too.

BLACK PEPPER. Add a pinch to 1 tablespoon aloe vera gel, and take three times a day with meals to relieve symptoms such as backache and abdominal pain. Aloe vera gel taken with a pinch of cumin works well, too.

CHERRIES. An Ayurvedic remedy to relieve PMS symptoms, including bloating and mood swings, is to eat 10 fresh cherries on an empty stomach each day for one week before the start of the menstrual period.

CHICKEN. It's rich in Vitamin B6, which may be depleted in women who suffer from PMS. Vitamin B6 may help relieve depression by raising levels of serotonin, a mood-enhancer, in the brain. Other B6-rich foods include fish, milk, brown rice, whole grains, soybeans, beans, walnuts, and green leafy vegetables.

CINNAMON. Good sleep habits are important in the treatment of PMS, and a brew of cinnamon tea is relaxing just before bed. Sweeten to taste with honey. Chamomile tea is a relaxing bedtime choice, too.

OATMEAL. It breaks down slowly and gradually releases sugar into the bloodstream. This slow, steady release combats the craving that comes with PMS. Rye bread, pasta, basmati rice, and fruit produce the same effect.

PASTA. This is enriched with magnesium, which is important for normal hormonal function. A lack of magnesium may be the cause of muscle cramps. Other magnesium-rich foods include green vegetables, breakfast cereals (skip those sugary ones), and potatoes.

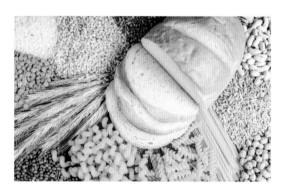

SUNFLOWER SEEDS. They're rich in omega-6 fatty acid, which may be missing in women who suffer with PMS. Pumpkin and sesame seeds are also rich in it.

TURKEY. It supplies tryptophan, an amino acid that converts into serotonin, a mood-enhancer. Cottage cheese is another source of tryptophan.

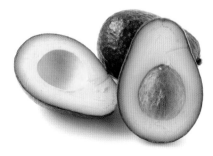

MORE DO'S & DON'TS

- **Forgo fats.** They may make PMS symptoms worse. Limit fat to less than 20 percent of your daily calories. Here's how to do the math:

  1. Divide your average daily calories by 5: If you eat 2,000 calories a day, that's 400.

  2. Divide that by 9. There are 9 calories per gram of fat: That comes to about 44 grams of fat allowed each day.

- Crunch on carbs. Fresh fruits, vegetables, and whole-grain cereals and breads can reduce the cravings that come with PMS. They also help elevate mood. Eat smaller meals, then snack on these carbohydrates every three hours: popcorn (skip the butter), pretzels, rice cakes. Consume about 100 calories per snack.

- Cut the caffeine. And that goes for coffee, cola, and chocolate. Caffeine contributes to breast pain and anxiety, two of the leading PMS complaints.

SUPPLEMENTS WITH A PMS PUNCH

Studies show that symptoms of PMS may be relieved by certain vitamin and mineral supplements. Check with your doctor before you take any of these. They all can have serious side effects.

VITAMIN/MINERAL	DAILY DOSAGE
Vitamin E	400 IU
Vitamin B6	50-100 milligrams
Calcium citrate	1,000 milligrams
Magnesium	300-500 milligrams

DON'T DO DIURETICS

Feeling a little bloated? Are your ankles puffed up enough to make three instead of two? Bloat and water retention are common symptoms of PMS, but avoid the common cure-all diuretics. They can wash away essential minerals, such as potassium, that are helpful in fighting PMS symptoms. (Heart palpitations can be a PMS side effect, and potassium evens out heart rhythm.) Instead, try natural diuretics such as parsley or dandelion tea or fresh, steamed asparagus. Limit salt and alcohol intake, too.

SEASONAL AFFECTIVE DISORDER

Ho hum. Another day, so much to do. But you can't seem to drag yourself out of bed. In fact, with Ma in her kerchief and Pa in his cap, the only thing you'd really like to do is snuggle in between the covers for your long winter's nap.

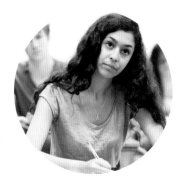

If that's a description of the way you feel every winter, you could be suffering from seasonal affective disorder, or SAD. It's a poorly understood condition that affects some people during the winter months, when there is less sunlight.

In addition to a depressed mood, symptoms of SAD include cravings for carbohydrates, inability to concentrate, irritability, lethargy, weight gain, and a lack of interest in sex.

Although the link between the gray, short days of winter and SAD is well-established, no one knows why some people are affected and others are not. Current thinking associates SAD with too much melatonin, the hormone that causes you to be sleepy. Normally, sunlight stops melatonin production in the body, and darkness starts it. When adequate sunlight is missing, as it usually is in the winter months, that wanna-go-to-sleep hormone kicks into overtime production because there's nothing around to tell it to turn itself off. Some medical researchers compare SAD to hibernation. During the winter, many animals store up on the carbohydrates, crawl into a cozy cave, resist the mating urge, and snooze until spring. Sounds pretty primal, but that's exactly the way people who suffer SAD react, only in a modified version.

Another theory is that SAD is a result of a delay in the timing of the body clock. In SAD patients, the body's lowest temperature occurs at 6 A.M., rather than at 3 A.M. as it should normally. As a result, they are awakening when physiologically it is the middle of the night. When treated with light from 6 A.M. to 8 A.M., these patients experience a shift in minimum temperature to an earlier time and an associated shift in mood.

Doctors often treat SAD with antidepressants. For some, they work. For others, the side effects are overwhelming, often worse than the SAD itself. So if you've got SAD, look in the kitchen for some relief.

KITCHEN CURES

APRICOTS. This fruit gradually raises serotonin levels and helps keep them there, as do apples, pears, grapes, plums, grapefruits, and oranges.

AVOCADOS. They are high in natural serotonin, which seems to suppress appetite. Also high in natural serotonin are dates, bananas, plums, eggplant, papayas, passion fruit, plantains, pineapples, and tomatoes.

BASMATI RICE. The sugar in this rice is slow to release into the bloodstream, which helps blood sugar levels stay constant instead of going through highs and lows. Drastic changes in blood sugar can lead to weight gain, which is a side effect of SAD. Other foods with a similar effect on blood sugar are rye bread and pasta.

BOUILLON. When the carbohydrate craving is just about to defeat you, drink some hot bouillon or broth. Hot liquids in the belly are filling, and consuming them before a meal is an old diet trick that reduces food consumption. Better the bouillon than the banana cream pie.

CEREALS. Cooked cereal, unsweetened muesli, and bran flakes are slow to release sugar into the bloodstream, which helps raise serotonin levels.

COTTAGE CHEESE. It's high in tryptophan, which is lacking in people with SAD. Other foods just as high in tryptophan are turkey, fish, and eggs.

HERBAL TEAS. Any herbal tea is a better choice than teas with caffeine. Your reduced energy level may cause you to turn to caffeine for a boost, but it can also cause anxiety, muscle tension, and stomach problems, so opt for herbal. Chamomile, peppermint, and cinnamon are pleasant-tasting choices. Drink a cup instead of giving in to your carbohydrate cravings.

LEGUMES. These help maintain an even serotonin level throughout the day and night.

SHELLFISH. These are high in tyrosine, which forms chemicals that act on the brain cells to improve concentration and alertness, both of which become sluggish with SAD. Other foods high in tyrosine are fish, chicken, skinless turkey, cottage cheese, plain yogurt, skim milk, eggs, tofu, and very lean ham, pork, and lamb.

TURKEY. Protein foods such as turkey, low fat cottage cheese, chicken, and low fat dairy products can reduce the carbohydrate cravings of SAD as well as control the weight gain that occurs during SAD months.

BAD SAD FOODS

Because overeating and weight gain often go hand-in-hand with SAD, you need to take extra care to avoid the foods that trigger carbohydrate cravings. **Here's a list of some of the worst offenders and what they do:**

- Sweets: Sugar, honey, soft drinks, cookies, candy, cake. These quickly raise blood sugar levels and provide a quick serotonin boost that falls off rapidly. When this happens, the brain wants another quick fix and you crave more. This can turn into a never-ending cycle, since the body wants a serotonin high all the time.

- Simple Carbohydrates: Bread, bagel, potatoes. Starchy foods also cause a rapid rise in blood sugar, which gives the brain its fast serotonin high, then drops you like a rock.

- Fats: Butter, margarine, oil, and fatty foods. These can cause the weight gain that accompanies SAD. Weight gain may also contribute to the depression associated with SAD.

SORE THROAT

It's scratchy, tender, and swollen, and you dread the simple task of swallowing. But you must swallow, and when you do, you brace yourself for the unavoidable pain. If you've got a sore throat, you're in good company; everybody gets them, and 40 million people trek to the doctor's office for treatment of one every year.

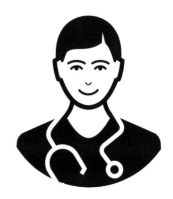

The mechanics of a sore throat are pretty simple. It's an inflammation of the pharynx, which is the tube that extends from the back of the mouth to the esophagus. **The following are the leading causes of sore throat:**

- Viral infection (colds, flu, etc.). Often accompanied by fever, achy muscles, and runny nose, viral infections can't be cured but their symptoms can be treated. A sore throat from a viral source will generally disappear on its own within several days.

- Bacterial infection, especially from a streptococcal bacteria (strep throat). Symptoms are much like those of a viral infection but may be more severe and long lasting. Often a bacterial infection is accompanied by headache, stomachache, and swollen glands in the neck. A strep infection is generally treated with antibiotics because permanent heart or kidney damage can result. Culturing the bacteria is the only way a doctor can determine the cause of the sore throat.

While those are the primary reasons for a sore throat, there are others, including:

- Smoking
- Acid reflux
- Allergies
- Dry air, especially at night when you may sleep with your mouth open
- Mouth breathing

- Throat abuse: singing, shouting, coughing
- Polyps or cancer
- Infected tonsils
- Food allergy

Whatever the cause, you want a cure when your throat's on fire. In some cases, medical attention is definitely required to cure the underlying infection. But there are soothing remedies to be found in the kitchen that can stand alone or work side-by-side with traditional medicine to stifle that soreness.

KITCHEN CURES

CIDER VINEGAR. This sore throat cure is found in several different remedies. Here are a few of the more popular ones:

For sipping: Mix 1 tablespoon each of honey and cider vinegar in 1 cup warm water.

For gargling: You'll need 1 teaspoon salt, $\frac{1}{2}$ cup cider vinegar, and 1 cup warm water. Dissolve the salt in the vinegar, then mix in the water. Gargle every 15 minutes as necessary.

CINNAMON. Mix 2 parts cinnamon, 2 parts ginger, and 3 parts licorice powder. Steep 1 teaspoon of this mixture in 1 cup boiling water for ten minutes, then drink as a sore throat cure three times a day.

GARLIC. This Amish remedy can treat or prevent sore throats. Peel a fresh clove, slice it in half, and place 1 piece in each cheek. Suck on the garlic like a cough drop. Occasionally, crush your teeth against the garlic, not to bite it in half, but to release its allicin, a chemical that can kill the bacteria that causes strep.

HORSERADISH. Try this Russian sore throat cure. Combine 1 tablespoon pure horseradish or horseradish root with 1 teaspoon honey and 1 teaspoon ground cloves. Mix in a glass of warm water and drink slowly.

LEMON JUICE. Mix 1 tablespoon each of honey and lemon juice in 1 cup warm water. Sip this mixture.

LIME JUICE. Combine 1 spoonful with a spoonful of honey and take as often as needed for a sore throat.

MARJORAM. Make a soothing tea with a spoonful of marjoram steeped in a cup of boiling water for ten minutes. Strain, then sweeten to taste with honey.

ONIONS. This tear-promoting veggie contains allicin, which can kill the bacteria that causes strep. Eat them raw or sautéed.

PEPPERMINT OIL. Add 2 drops each of peppermint and eucalyptus oils to 2 teaspoons olive oil and massage on the throat and upper chest for a nice, relaxing throat-soother.

SAGE. This curative herb is a great sore throat gargle. Mix 1 teaspoon in 1 cup boiling water. Steep for ten minutes, then strain. Add 1 teaspoon each cider vinegar and honey, then gargle four times a day.

TURMERIC. Try this gargle to calm a cranky throat. Mix together 1 cup hot water, $\frac{1}{2}$ teaspoon turmeric, and $\frac{1}{2}$ teaspoon salt. Gargle with the mixture twice a day. If you're not good with the gargle, mix $\frac{1}{2}$ teaspoon turmeric in 1 cup hot milk and drink. Turmeric stains clothing, so be careful when mixing and gargling.

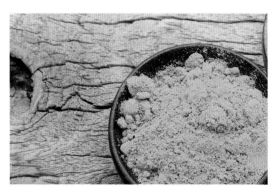

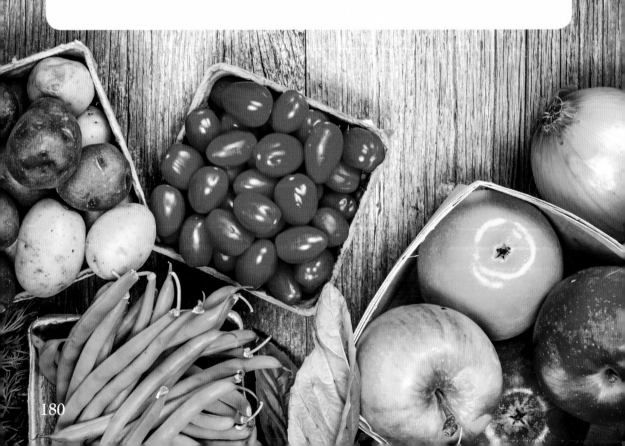

HERBAL CURES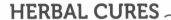

Chamomile. Make a tea by adding 1 teaspoon chamomile to 1 cup boiling water. Steep for ten minutes, strain, then gargle three to four times a day.

Make a poultice by mixing 1 tablespoon chamomile flowers in 2 cups boiling water. Steep five minutes, then strain. Soak a clean towel in the warm solution, wring it out, and apply to throat. Remove when cold and reapply as often as necessary.

Horehound. This is a great remedy for sore throats, but it's not a common herb found on most shelves. If you do happen to find it, make a tea with 1 tablespoon horehound leaves and 1 cup boiling water. Steep, strain, and gargle. Or, suck on some horehound hard candy.

STOMACH UPSET

You and the wife celebrated your promotion with dinner at your
favorite barbecue joint. You've been working hard for months,
you think, so you deserve to cut loose a little. On the way home
you groan and mutter that you wish you had stopped after that
first barbecue platter. Your wife shrugs her shoulders. You both
know the price for your revelry will be a painful night of bloating, gas, and heartburn.

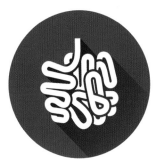

But sometimes your tummy can turn on you even when you haven't
been making one too many trips to the buffet table. It's important to
know what's normal tummy trouble and what's something to take more seriously.

THE DIGESTIVE DANCE

When you eat something, the digestive process begins right away in your mouth. Your
salivary glands produce digestive juices that lubricate your food and prepare fat for digestion.
The food travels through your esophagus into your stomach, where digestive juices continue
to break food down even further so it can travel on to the small intestine. The pancreas and
liver secrete other digestive juices that flow into the small intestines. In the small intestine,
vital nutrients including vitamins, minerals, water, salt, carbohydrates, and proteins are
sucked out of the food and absorbed into your body. By the time your dinner makes its way
to the large intestines, it's mostly bulk and water. The large intestines absorb the water and
help you get rid of the, umm, excess.

But sometimes things in the digestive system go awry and cause indigestion, a catchall term
that means you simply have trouble digesting your food. When you eat too much, or you eat
the wrong foods, you may get one of a number of indigestion symptoms mentioned above:
nausea, vomiting, heartburn, bloating, or gas.

Those unpleasant feelings may send you running to the drugstore for relief, and if they do,
you've got plenty of company. The American Gastroenterological Association says that
digestive problems are one of the most common reasons Americans take over-the-counter
medications. Indigestion can be a symptom of something more serious, such as gastritis, an
ulcer, severe heartburn, irritable bowel syndrome, or diverticulitis. But if it's just the result of
over-doing it at dinner, try some of these kitchen cures for relief.

KITCHEN CURES

APPLE. Adding fiber to your diet will help alleviate stomachaches and keep your digestive system healthy. One study of fiber's effect on the tummy discovered that people who ate fiber-rich foods at the first sign of a tummyache cut their chances of getting a full-blown upset stomach in half. If you haven't been eating much fiber, be sure to start slowly. Jumping in with loads of fiber-rich foods after living on burgers and fries will give you a mean case of gas. Add fiber gradually over a few months and drink plenty of water to avoid overloading your system. To get started, grab an apple and nosh away, but remember to eat the peel—that's where you get most of your roughage.

BANANA. If you have a sensitive tummy, bland foods such as bananas seem to ease the pain. One study found that half the people who took banana powder capsules every day for two months eased their tummy pain. You can get similar results by eating a banana—or better yet a plantain banana—every day.

CARAWAY SEEDS. These seeds act very similarly to fennel seeds. They help with digestion and gas. You can either make a tea from the seed or you can do what people in Middle Eastern countries have done for centuries—simply chew on the seeds after dinner. Caraway seed tea: Place 1 teaspoon caraway seeds in a cup and add boiling water.

Cover the cup and let stand for ten minutes. Strain well and drink up to 3 cups a day—be sure to drink on an empty stomach.

CINNAMON. This aromatic spice stimulates the digestive system, helping things move along the digestive tract smoothly. You can make a cinnamon tea by stirring $\frac{1}{4}$ to $\frac{1}{2}$ teaspoon cinnamon powder into 1 cup hot water. Let the tea stand for up to five minutes and drink.

CRACKERS. You haven't eaten anything all day, and you can't understand why your stomach is churning and burning. The answer is probably overactive stomach acids. And your best bet is to eat something but to stick with something bland, such as nibbling on crackers.

FENNEL SEEDS. This remedy is one of the most prescribed for gas and stomach cramps by medical herbalists. Try a fennel tea for your stomach: Place 1 teaspoon fennel seeds in a cup and add boiling water. Cover the cup and let stand for ten minutes. Strain well and drink up to 3 cups a day—be sure to drink on an empty stomach.

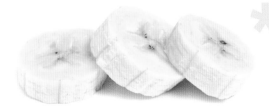

GINGER. Ginger is a long-time helper for stomach ailments of all types—particularly nausea and gas. Ginger helps food flow smoothly through the digestive tract, allowing the body to better absorb nutrients. Drink a cup of ginger tea to get your stomach back on track. To make your own ginger tea: Add $1/2$ teaspoon ground ginger to a cup of hot water, let stand for up to three minutes, strain, and drink away.

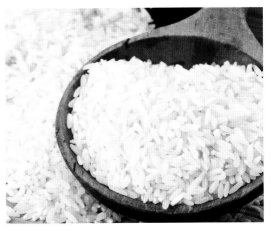

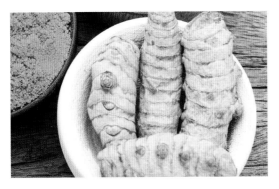

MINT. A folk remedy for indigestion, mint (in the form of peppermint or spearmint) can soothe a troubled tummy. Mint helps food move through the intestines properly and eases stomach cramps. **Sip a cup of mint tea to let the herb work its magic:** Put 1 teaspoon dried mint in a cup and add boiling water. Cover the cup and let it stand for ten minutes. Strain and drink up to 3 cups of the warm tea a day. Be sure to drink it on an empty stomach.

RICE. If an overflow of stomach acid bothers you, try eating $1/2$ cup cooked rice with your dinner. It's a complex carbohydrate that keeps the stomach busy churning, diverting excess acid. Plus it's a bland food that tends to be easy on the stomach.

SODA POP. Sipping on a can of decaffeinated soda can help settle your stomach. This trick is especially useful if you've eaten too much. The carbonation in the soda causes you to burp, which is the quickest way to get relief from an overfull belly.

THYME. Thyme stimulates the digestive tract, helps with stomach cramping, and relieves gas pressure. Try some thyme in a bottle (or cup) for your tummy trouble: Place 1 teaspoon dried thyme leaves in a cup. Fill the cup with boiling water and let stand, covered, for ten minutes. Strain and drink on an empty stomach up to three times a day.

MORE DO'S AND DON'TS

- Think twice about milk. Though many people think milk can soothe an aching tummy, it actually may do more harm than good. People who are lactose intolerant have trouble digesting milk and end up with bloating, gas, and cramping.

- Cut the coffee. Coffee causes stomach irritation in some people.

- Ax the alcohol. Alcohol is also a stomach irritant. If you have a sensitive tummy, skip the after-dinner drink.

- Pass on pepper. Red or black pepper may add a kick to food, but it can also kick you in the tummy. Avoid it if it bothers your stomach.

- Choose produce carefully. Some vegetables and fruits are notorious for their ability to produce tummy trouble. Watch out for broccoli, cabbage, Brussels sprouts, and melons.

- Wash your beans. Beans are the "musical fruit," but you can take the music out of them. Let them soak overnight in water, then drain the water and replace it with fresh water before cooking. Rinse canned beans, too. This simple technique will help avert gassy problems.

- Eat up. Don't skip meals. It allows acid to build up in your stomach and can leave you with an aching tummy.

FOODS MOST LIKELY
TO CAUSE TUMMY TROUBLE

German researchers wanted to know what foods caused the most trouble for people. So they asked people what foods tended to create an aching tummy. The top three offenders for normal, healthy eaters were mayonnaise, cabbage, and fried and salted foods.

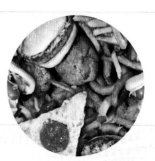

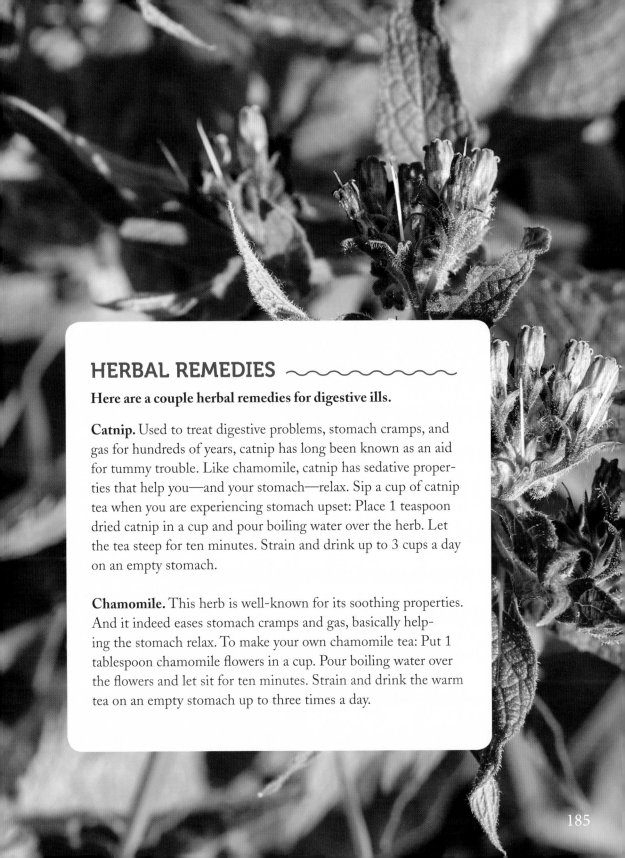

HERBAL REMEDIES

Here are a couple herbal remedies for digestive ills.

Catnip. Used to treat digestive problems, stomach cramps, and gas for hundreds of years, catnip has long been known as an aid for tummy trouble. Like chamomile, catnip has sedative properties that help you—and your stomach—relax. Sip a cup of catnip tea when you are experiencing stomach upset: Place 1 teaspoon dried catnip in a cup and pour boiling water over the herb. Let the tea steep for ten minutes. Strain and drink up to 3 cups a day on an empty stomach.

Chamomile. This herb is well-known for its soothing properties. And it indeed eases stomach cramps and gas, basically helping the stomach relax. To make your own chamomile tea: Put 1 tablespoon chamomile flowers in a cup. Pour boiling water over the flowers and let sit for ten minutes. Strain and drink the warm tea on an empty stomach up to three times a day.

ULCERS

It's only in the last decade that scientific evidence conclusively proved that ulcers are most often caused by a bacterial infection, not by the Type-A, pressure-cooker personality that was the subject of countless jokes. Misconceptions and myths die hard, though, so there are some people who haven't gotten the word yet and still believe that the demanding boss or the overachiever are more likely to work themselves into an ulcer. While these personality characteristics may aggravate an existing ulcer (not to mention the people they associate with), they don't cause one.

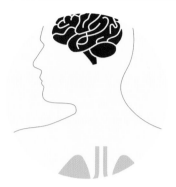

THERE'S A HOLE IN THE BUCKET

An ulcer is a sore or hole in the protective mucosal lining of the gastrointestinal tract. Ulcers appear in the area of the stomach or the duodenum, the upper part of the small intestine, where caustic digestive juices, pepsin, and hydrochloric acid are present. Today we know that the majority of ulcers are the result of an infection with a bacteria called Helicobacter pylori (*H. pylori*). This bacteria makes the stomach and small intestine more susceptible to the erosive effects of the digestive juices. The bacteria may also cause the stomach to produce more acid.

There are some lifestyle factors that can contribute to the development of an ulcer. These include alcohol consumption, eating and drinking foods that contain caffeine, significant physical (not emotional) stress such as severe burns and major surgery, and excessive use of certain over-the-counter pain medications such as aspirin or ibuprofen. Studies have shown that smoking also tends to increase the chances of developing an ulcer, slows the healing of existing ulcers, and makes a recurrence more likely. Family history of ulcers also appears to play a role in susceptibility.

WHO GETS ULCERS?

If Type-A folks don't automatically get ulcers, then who does? The cause lies less in personality and more in stomach makeup. Researchers believe some people just produce more stomach acid than others. If stomach acid production isn't the problem, then a weak stomach may be. The stomach lining in certain individuals may be less able to withstand the onslaught of gastric acids. Lifestyle factors mentioned above can also weaken the stomach's lining.

SIGNS AND SYMPTOMS

You're probably familiar with the most typical symptom of a brewing ulcer: a burning or gnawing pain between the breastbone and navel. This pain is more common between meals (it improves with eating but returns a few hours later) and in the middle of the night or toward dawn.

Less typical symptoms include nausea or vomiting, weight loss and loss of appetite, and frequent burping or bloating.

If you have an ulcer or suspect you may have one, you should be under the care of a physician. But between visits to the doctor, there are ways to care for your digestive tract.

KITCHEN CURES

BANANAS. These fruits contain an antibacterial substance that may inhibit the growth of ulcer-causing *H. pylori*. And studies show that animals fed bananas have a thicker stomach wall and greater mucus production in the stomach, which helps build a better barrier between digestive acids and the lining of the stomach. Eating plantains is also helpful.

CABBAGE. Researchers have found that ulcer patients who drink 1 quart of raw cabbage juice a day can often heal their ulcers in five days. If chugging a quart of cabbage juice turns your stomach inside out, researchers also found that those who eat plain cabbage have quicker healing times as well. Time for some coleslaw!

CAYENNE PEPPER. Used moderately, a little cayenne pepper can go a long way in helping ulcers. The pepper stimulates blood flow to bring nutrients to the stomach. To make a cup of peppered tea, mix 1/4 teaspoon cayenne pepper in 1 cup hot water. Drink a cup a day. A dash of cayenne pepper can also be added to soups, meats, and other savory dishes.

GARLIC. Garlic's antibacterial properties include fighting *H. pylori*. Take two small crushed cloves a day.

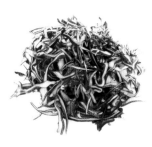

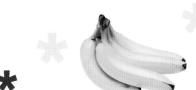

LICORICE. Several modern studies have demonstrated the ulcer-healing abilities of licorice. Licorice does its part not by reducing stomach acid but rather by reducing the ability of stomach acid to damage stomach lining. Properties in licorice encourage digestive mucosal tissues to protect themselves from acid. Licorice can be used in encapsulated form, but for a quick cup of licorice tea, cut 1 ounce licorice root into slices and cover with 1 quart boiling water. Steep, cool, and strain. (If licorice root is unavailable, cut 1 ounce licorice sticks into slices.) You can also try licorice candy if it's made with real licorice (the label will say "licorice mass") and not just flavored with anise. Don't eat more than 1 ounce per day.

PLUMS. Red- and purple-colored foods inhibit the growth of *H. pylori*. Like plums, berries too can help you fight the good fight.

RABBIT FOOD?

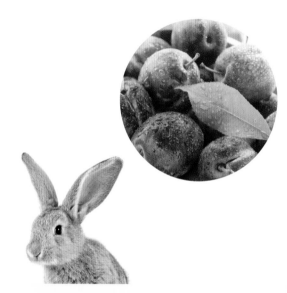

- Be like a bunny and nibble throughout the day. The key to keeping gastric juices from attacking the digestive tract lining is to keep them busy with food. Snacking on healthy treats, such as carrot sticks and whole-wheat crackers, should do the trick. Also, consider becoming a six-small-meals-a-day type person rather than a three-meals-a-day type.

FOOD SURPRISES

Milk was an early treatment for ulcer flare-ups, but it is no longer considered a good drink if you have ulcers. Foods high in calcium, such as milk, stimulate stomach acid. Limit your milk intake according to your doctor's advice.

Highly spiced and fried foods, on the other hand, once were thought to be prime culprits in starting ulcers. But research has shown that they have little or no bearing either on the development or the course of an ulcer. This is not to say that such food won't cause irritation.

Watch what you pull from the refrigerator and note your gut reaction to each. If you experience discomfort, ban the food from the fridge. If nothing happens after popping that pizza slice into your pouch—rejoice and enjoy!

URINARY TRACT INFECTION

You stand in front of the bathroom door for the twentieth time in the last hour. You've got to go, but every time you do, you end up with only a painful trickle. You recognize the burning sensation that makes every trip to the toilet an ordeal. You've got a urinary tract infection. Urinary tract infections (UTIs) are the second most common reason people visit their doctors each year. Men get UTIs, but they are much more common in women—more than eight million women head to their doctor for UTI treatment annually. And 20 percent of these women will get a second UTI.

If you've ever had a UTI, you'll probably never forget the symptoms. It usually starts with a sudden and frequent need to visit the potty. When you get there, you can squeeze out only a little bit of urine, and that's usually accompanied by a burning sensation in your bladder and/ or urethra. In more extreme cases you may end up with fever, chills, back pain, and even blood in your urine.

UTIs that last longer than two days require medical intervention. Untreated UTIs can infect the kidneys and turn into a much more serious problem. To help prevent a UTI from developing or nip one in the bud, try some of the remedies available in your own kitchen.

KITCHEN CURES

BLUEBERRIES. Blueberries and cranberries are from the same plant family and seem to have the same bacteria-inhibiting properties. In one study, blueberry juice was found to prevent UTIs. Since you're not likely to find a gallon of blueberry juice at your local store, try sprinkling a handful of these flavorful, good-for-you berries over your morning cereal.

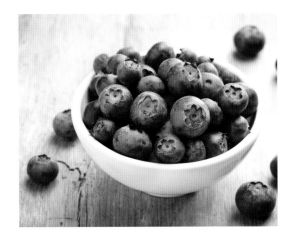

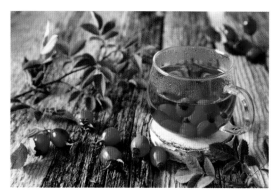

PINEAPPLE. Bromelain is an enzyme found in pineapples. In one study, people with a UTI who were given bromelain along with their usual round of antibiotics got rid of their infection. Only half the people who were given a placebo plus an antibiotic showed no signs of lingering infection. Eating a cup of pineapple tastes good and may just help rid you of your infection.

CRANBERRY JUICE. Many studies have found that drinking cranberry juice may help you avoid urinary tract infections. It appears that cranberry juice prevents infection-causing bacteria from bedding down in your bladder, and it also has a very mild antibiotic affect. Drinking as little as 4 ounces of cranberry juice a day can help keep your bladder infection-free. But if you tend to get UTIs or are dealing with one right now, try to drink at least 2 to 4 glasses of cranberry juice a day. If pure cranberry juice is just too bitter for your taste buds, you can substitute cranberry juice cocktail. It seems to have the same effect as the pure stuff. **Take note:** If you have a UTI, cranberry juice is not a replacement for doctor-prescribed antibiotics in treating your infection.

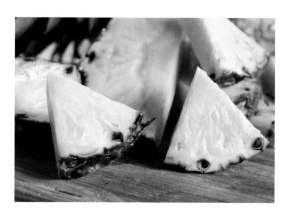

VITAMIN C. Some doctors are prescribing at least 5,000 mg or more of vitamin C a day for patients who develop recurrent urinary tract infections. Vitamin C keeps the bladder healthy by acidifying the urine, essentially putting up a no-trespassing sign for potentially harmful bacteria.

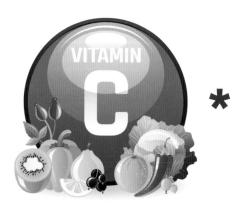

YEAST INFECTION

It's not a topic that comes up in polite conversation, and on the odd occasion that it does, it's approached in a whisper. No one wants to talk about a yeast infection, and no one wants to admit they have one. That's probably because it's known as one of those "personal" things that only affects women.

Well, in most cases that's true, but yeast infections are not restricted to women only. You know that diaper rash covering the cutest little bottom you've ever seen? Guess what? Yeast. And that condition called thrush that babies often develop in the mouth? Yeast again. So you see, yeast is not just about an unpleasant vaginal infection that no one wants to talk about. It's a fungus that can proliferate anywhere the breeding ground is right. And the breeding ground is right in the genital and oral areas because that's where *Candida albicans*, the fungus that causes a yeast infection, lives.

Yeast happens when the acidity of normal fluids is altered. Usually they're acidic enough to keep the yeast from flourishing. But when something goes wrong, the balance is tipped and the yeast have a party, multiplying over and over. What causes the imbalance? **Here are common factors:**

- Weakened immune system
- Diabetes
- Overuse of antibiotics
- Steroids
- In vaginal yeast infections, there may be additional factors:
- Hormonal changes, such as those that occur at puberty, pregnancy, or menopause
- Inadequate vaginal lubrication during intercourse
- Soap sensitivity
- Feminine hygiene deodorants and douches
- Spermicides

Yeast infections also can be transmitted between sexual partners. Using condoms or abstaining from sex during the infection are the best ways to prevent spreading it.

Typical symptoms of a vaginal yeast infection include intense itching and soreness accompanied by a thick white discharge. Symptoms of a genital yeast infection in men include irritation and itching in the genital area, sometimes accompanied by white discharge under the foreskin and/or swelling at the end of the penis. In the throat, yeast looks like creamy white patches.

Most yeast infections can be cured with remedies found on the pharmacy shelf either in cream or suppository form. There are also prescription medications available that will stop the problem in as little as three days. But, there are also simple kitchen panaceas that can bring relief or cure and even stop the disease from recurring.

KITCHEN CURES

BASIL. For thrush, make a basil tea and use it as a gargle. Boil 3 ½ cups water, remove from heat, and add 1 ¼ teaspoons ground basil. Cover and steep for 30 minutes. Cool and gargle. Or sweeten to taste with maple syrup and drink 1 cup twice a day.

CRANBERRY JUICE. Drunk unsweetened, it may acidify vaginal secretions and equip them to fight off the yeast.

GARLIC. Eating 2 fresh garlic cloves a day, either plain or minced and tossed in a salad or sauce, may prevent yeast infections or help clear up a case of thrush. Garlic has antifungal properties.

ROSEMARY. To relieve itching and burning, make a tea of rosemary, and use it as a douche or dab it onto the external area.

THYME. Make a thyme tea using 1 teaspoon dried thyme per 1 cup boiling water. Steep and drink 1 to 4 cups per day if you have a yeast infection.

YOGURT. The live culture in plain yogurt is a great remedy for a yeast infection, helping to restore the acid-bacteria balance in more ways than one.

THE NO-NO FOOD LIST

Certain foods can contribute to conditions that give rise to a yeast infection. If you are prone to getting the infection or already have one, **here are the foods to avoid:**

- Sugars, including white and brown sugar, honey, and molasses. Yeast feeds on sugar, so if you're prone to getting an infection, reduce the amount you eat. And during an infection, cut down further.

- Unrefined starches, such as refined pasta and white bread. Cut back if you're prone to getting yeast infections, and cut them out entirely when you have one. During the digestive process, unrefined starches break down into simple sugar.

- Alcohol. Those little *Candida albicans* really love the booze. It breaks down easily into sugar.

- Yeast and fermented foods, including breads and beer.

- Molds, including aged cheeses, mushrooms, dried fruits, fruit juice (unless it's fresh), peanuts, and peanut butter.